A LITTLE BIT

OF

YOGA

A LITTLE BIT
OF
YOGA

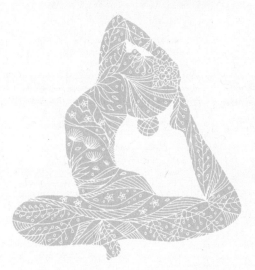

AN INTRODUCTION TO
POSTURES & PRACTICE

MEAGAN STEVENSON

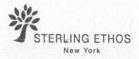

STERLING ETHOS
New York

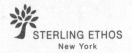

STERLING ETHOS
New York

An Imprint of Sterling Publishing
1166 Avenue of the Americas
New York, NY 10036

Text © 2018 Meagan Stevenson
Cover © 2018 Sterling Publishing Co., Inc.

ISBN 978-1-4549-3226-0

Distributed in Canada by Sterling Publishing Co., Inc.
c/o Canadian Manda Group, 664 Annette Street
Toronto, Ontario M6S 2C8, Canada
Distributed in the United Kingdom by GMC Distribution Services
Castle Place, 166 High Street, Lewes, East Sussex BN7 1XU, England
Distributed in Australia by NewSouth Books
University of South Wales, Sydney, NSW 2052, Australia

For information about custom editions, special sales, and premium and corporate purchases, please
contact Sterling Special Sales at 800-805-5489 or specialsales@sterlingpublishing.com.

Manufactured in the United States of America

2 4 6 8 10 9 7 5 3 1

sterlingpublishing.com

Interior design by Shannon Nicole Plunkett
Cover design by Elizabeth Mihaltse Lindy

Image Credits
Shutterstock (cover, throughout): Benjavisa Ruangvaree (body); satit_srihin (border)

CONTENTS

INTRODUCTION

Three years ago, I had an afternoon off from my crazy work schedule. It was summer in Brooklyn, a particularly hot one at that, and I was craving a yoga class but didn't want to leave my neighborhood. Wandering the streets of Stuyvesant Heights, I remembered a yoga studio a few blocks away in a giant brownstone. On a whim, I signed up for an early-evening class. For whatever reason, at that particular time in my life, on that particular day, I remember feeling unbelievably empowered as soon as the class began. With each pose, I felt my body surging with energy. I felt excited to be in that space, present and looking forward to what move would come next. I remember holding warrior 2 and feeling as if I could conquer anything in my life, big or small. The studio was tucked away in a cozy home. The summer golden hour beamed gently into the space and melted away as the class went on—no mirrors, no distractions. It was the first time in my entire life that I took a class just because I truly LOVED yoga, and in this magical brownstone I found confidence in my practice.

We spend hours of our life at the gym, in classes, sweating and moving because we're told we must if we want a great "summer body," or we are guilted into it because it's what we "have" to do to look good. Figuring out what gets you excited to carve an hour out of your day is what excites me: choosing to do yoga not because you need to work out, but because your soul needs it, your mind needs it, your body wants to move in that way. It is a privilege to get to move together, as a community and as an individual. Find what helps you celebrate being alive, with the ability to take the deepest inhales and deepest exhales possible. My wish is for each and every person who reads this book to find their own personal yoga haven that makes every fiber of their existence feel invigorated to live on this planet.

❈ 1 ❈

YOGA
MYTHS

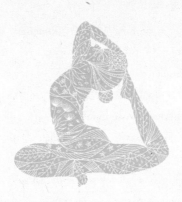

"The success is of yoga does not lie in the ability to perform postures but in how it positively changes the way we live our lives and our relationships."

—T. K. V. DESIKACHAR

I'M NOT FLEXIBLE."

"I'm not good at it."

"It's too expensive."

"I'm unsure if I'm doing it right."

"I don't know where to begin."

"Everyone else looks like a pretzel and I can't even touch my toes."

"I'm worried people will judge me."

"I'm worried I'll judge myself."

If I had a dollar for every time I'd invited a friend, coworker, or new aquaintance to take my yoga class and the first thing out of their mouth was fear or insecurity, I'd have enough money to live in New York *lavishly*.

When trying something new, our immediate reaction is often to talk ourselves out of it. Maybe we make a New Year's resolution. Insert excuse number one, then time passes. It occurs to us to try again—cue excuse number two, then more time passes. By the time you've come around to excuse number three, it's the end of the year and it's time to make a new resolution. What excuse will continue to keep you from trying yoga? Is it fear of the unknown? Like dipping your toe into the pool to check the temperature first, there's hesitation, a sense of worry, a gut reaction of fear. The water is just fine, and the more you put off taking the plunge, the more time you waste not enjoying the swim. I'm here to reassure you that it's worth the jump. Yoga is for *everyone*—no ifs, ands, or buts about it. There are many misconceptions about what yoga actually is and what it *has* to be. Here are some major misconceptions:

ONE HAS TO BE "FIT" OR "FLEXIBLE" TO DO YOGA.

Surprise! That's a major reason why we do yoga: to gain body awareness. Everyone starts as a beginner. Though it may seem like everyone is looking at the newbie in the back, they're one hundred percent more focused on their own bodies and selves than they are on judging you. There's no perfect "yoga body." Everyone is included, and all ages, shapes, sizes, and colors are welcome. If you encounter someone who tells you otherwise, make eye contact as you roll your mat out and flash a big smile. You should feel at home wherever you decide to practice. Allow yourself to enjoy the "firsts" of inviting yoga into your life. We rarely get to experience new things as adults, so let yourself give in to the bubbly feeling of a first.

DOING YOGA MEANS INCLUDING FANCY PHYSICAL POSES. Social media has morphed yoga into extravagant flows, incredible handstands, and seemingly impossible poses. While those are beautiful in their own ways, yoga is not just about the asanas. Eventually, you can work toward adding some fanciness to your flow . . . or maybe you continually keep it simple. Your practice is what you make it. Yoga can be sitting for a few minutes every morning connecting your breath to your body, moving between cat/cow and then taking child's pose, or simply lying in savasana tracking your breath; these all can be versions of yoga.

YOGA IS ONLY FOR WOMEN. Oh boy, this one is my favorite. I've had many men tell me they assume yoga is easy, just stretching, or that it is too "girly." Nothing is more satisfying than a boyfriend begrudgingly joining his girlfriend for yoga, and ending the class fully covered in sweat, looking at his lady and mouthing, "That was hard!" Sure, there's restorative flows that target release and relaxation, but a Vinyasa or Ashtanga will kick your butt in all the right ways when done correctly. Your core will be strengthened, your arms will be toned, your soul will be happy.

I'M NOT GOOD ENOUGH. Think about learning how to write for the first time. When you look at your handwriting from first grade and compare it to what you can do now, you'll notice quite a difference (I hope . . .). Over time, you acquired muscle memory. It didn't happen overnight, but throughout your life you've refined a simple movement and have maintained it by writing as often as you can. The same thing applies to yoga! The more you move through flows, the more your body adjusts and learns. "Good" and "bad" at yoga don't exist. Over time, you'll begin to build body awareness. Trust me. I spent a very small percentage of my middle school years playing volleyball and I was admittedly not great. Inherently, I had zero athletic ability and no desire to get sweaty, thus leading me to band and theater as suitable substitutes. The body awareness I've found over the last ten years is all from my own hard work. I can with confidence tell you that this isn't something that comes naturally to all, and that's okay! It's never too late to start yoga.

ALL YOGIS ARE HEALTH NUTS/ARE VEGAN/DON'T DRINK. Listen, I love pizza as much as I love yoga. When I say "it's all about balance," it truly is. Including yoga in my practice has made me more mindful of what I eat, but I don't restrict myself if I'd like to have a glass of wine on occasion. You can live your life and include a practice. You might be more inclined to choose broccoli over nachos post-class, but forcing a vegan lifestyle on yourself to be able to do yoga is one hundred percent not necessary.

Whew! Now that that's out of the way, let go of any other preconceived notions and leave them right here in chapter one. Your practice is what you make it. There are a million different perspectives, opinions, and celebrations of what yoga is. Take what resonates with you, and bring it to your mat.

WHAT IS IT THAT KEEPS YOU PERSONALLY FROM DOING YOGA?

Is it the price of classes? Perhaps it seems boring, or you took a class with a teacher that made it too serious, or not serious enough? Was it the studio itself, or maybe *om*ing just isn't your thing? When teaching class, I like to give my students tools to do yoga without me there, whether it be cuing what muscle groups should feel the strength and/or stretch in each movement, or the confidence to come into tree pose to find balance before a big interview. I'm going to load up your tool belt to help you start a little bit of yoga on your own, or perhaps to encourage you to find a space that feels right for you. A fully equipped yogi tool belt is key to finding confidence in yourself and your practice. Honor who you are, and find yoga that mirrors your soul.

ABANDONING YOUR FEAR

We've touched on the idea of judgment from others in the yoga room. No matter how grumpy the girl on the mat next to you looks, odds are she doesn't care what you're doing. When walking into class, if you feel as though you're personally watching everyone else and analyzing each skill level, that's a big sign that you do need some yoga in your life. I spent my first year of Bikram yoga constantly watching others. Not to learn, but in a self-deprecating way, thinking, "Wow, look at her balance. Will I ever have abs like that? Ugh, why can't I stretch my leg that high?! He is so still and focused. . . . Why can't I achieve that?" Questions like these attacked my mind every single time I tossed my towel over my mat, preparing for a ninety-minute sweatfest. I lived in constant fear that I wasn't good enough to be there.

My sophomore year of college, I was introduced to Kundalini yoga, a more intense type of yoga centered around heavy breathing (see more on page 17). While I don't practice it now, my eyes were opened wide to a completely different side of yoga. In fact, it was the polar opposite of what I'd always imagined "yoga" to be. No mirrors, same intensity, completely different feeling after class. My view of myself, my time in class, and my reason for doing yoga shifted drastically. The ability to judge myself less and my fear of being "bad" had slowly melted away. While it may take a while to shush those ever-present thoughts and fears, it's achievable. Maybe your fear is "What if I fall down or out of pose?" Guess what, it's inevitable! Even as an instructor I lose my balance. Finding space to grow from where you are and not being afraid to just be who you are on any given day when coming to class is what's important. The ability to confront your fears on your mat directly translates to how you confront your fears in everyday life, and that is an invaluable thing to take away from your practice.

❧ 2 ❧

WHAT IS
YOGA?

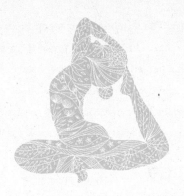

"Watch your thoughts; they become words. Watch your words; they become actions. Watch your actions; they become habits. Watch your habits; they become character. Watch your character; for it becomes your destiny."

—UNKNOWN

THE ROOTS OF WHAT WE KNOW AS "YOGA" RUN deep through Indian spiritual and religious practice. The word *yoga* has transformed over the course of many years to what we know today and has an extremely rich and complex story of its beginnings. There are many definitions of yoga, but the actual word means "union" or "connection." Basically, yoga is a way of connecting the body, mind, and breath as well as finding self-awareness. Connection to life, awareness of who we are and what we are is what

9

ties it all together. The term itself was found in ancient India's earliest script, the Vedas. This is the first use of the word *yoga* (referred to originally as an actual physical chariot), where the Vedic priests were known to be "ascetic," which is someone who practices self-discipline and avoids self-indulgence. There are five important time periods in the journey to what yoga has become today.

VEDIC PERIOD

The Vedas were the original holy writings of Brahmanism. They combined texts, songs, and mantras that all recognize a higher power, which is known as Vedic yoga. This is what we know as the most ancient teaching of yoga, spiritual development and the ability to broaden the mind through a ritualistic practice. Rishis, those who have discovered eternal truth and deep levels of mindfulness through periods of intense meditation, were their teachers. These yogis felt most inclined to live in secluded, serene, quiet places close to nature. (Quiet, secluded—reminds me of . . . yoga studios!)

PRE-CLASSICAL YOGA

The period of the Upanishads, which are Hindu religious texts written in Sanskrit expanding on the Vedas, is generally understood to have occurred between the years 500 and 200 BCE. The Upanishads make up two hundred scriptures on expanding the inner reality of being a brahman (member of the highest priestly caste in the Hindu system). The three big-ticket items from the Upanishads include the ultimate reality, the transcendent self, and the relationship between them. What we now know as "yoga" is vastly different than what the rishis and gurus laid out spiritually. However, there is much admiration that vibrates through modern yoga for the different paths of yoga created from the Upanishads. This period also includes the Bhagavad Gita, which expanded on the concept of putting the ego on the back burner to let actions speak for who you are and letting go of your body's cravings, temptations, and aversions to access freedom.

CLASSICAL YOGA

This period of yoga tends to be a hodgepodge of information, some ideas even conflicting. But we start to see some sort of structure emerge. Most notably, it's known as the creation period of Patanjali's yoga sutras. These defined the path of Raja yoga, which delves into a branch of yoga that emphasizes mental dedication and meditative practices. There are eight "limbs" to Raja yoga that lead the way toward enlightenment: yama, niyama, asana, pranayama, pratyahara, dharana, dhyana, and samadhi (see page 37 for more information). These ideals are still extremely relevant to what we understand yoga to be today.

POST-CLASSICAL

Influenced by Patanjali's sutras, this next phase of the yoga world moved toward working on the body to prolong life. The teachings of the Vedas shifted out of focus, and the physical body became the main vessel to achieve enlightenment. The exploration of the physical-mental-spiritual connection began to expand, creating Tantra yoga as well as Hatha. We're starting to approach the yoga you're probably familiar with. . . .

MODERN

Yoga moves west! In the early 1900s, yoga masters traveled to the Western world promoting their teachings, which gained major attention. At this point, Hatha was the most prominent, with Indian teachers carving the path to the yoga we are most familiar with now. It's evolved and transcended through time, absorbing many ideals, mantras, asanas, secrets of meditation, and all the contemporary variations that we enjoy today.

So next time you're habitually pressing back into downward dog, remember that layers upon layers of history go into that one simple pose. The practice of yoga isn't just the tea-drinking, yoga-pants-wearing lifestyle image we see so often today—it is the result of thousands of years' worth of study and all of the contemporary variations we enjoy all day.

Nowadays, when we hear the word yoga, there's crazy amounts of modernization attached to it. It's become so relevant to our society, not only for physical health but recognized as one of the best natural therapies, that we even dedicated a day to celebrating it—June 21st is "International Yoga Day." But ultimately, the word "yoga" in Sanskrit derives from the work yuj, which means uniting the individual and universal consciousness. In other words, the end game isn't just to do some poses and breathe. Yoga is meant to bring you back to your harmony, your truth, your joy, your existence, your ability to connect to the energy of the world around you. If even for a moment you find some sort of connection to the truest version of you, yoga has done its job. With constant stimulus, the modern world is in dire need of a disconnect from screens and deeper connection to a grounded version of ourselves.

The history of how yoga and how it came to its contemporary form speaks volumes about humanity. It speaks to how simply moving and breathing can heal your soul and press a reset button on your being. We're able to prolong our life the more we can tap into our truest, happiest, and fullest selves. It's in our nature to move freely, like when we were babies rolling around on the ground, or the moment you stretch your arms over your head when you wake up in the morning. Studies have showed that just fifteen minutes of yoga can increase your serotonin levels, resulting in a happier you. That's the whole point of this whole "living" thing, right?—to find some sort of happiness so the next time you habitually press back into down dog.

WHAT YOGA IS RIGHT FOR ME?

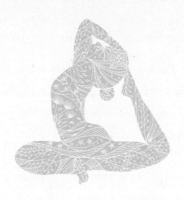

"Yoga is the perfect opportunity to be curious about who you are."
—JASON CRANDELL

I N THE LAST CHAPTER WE TRAVELED THROUGH THE
time periods in which different kinds of yoga developed. Now
we'll go through each type of yoga, exploring major benefits
that should help you decide which is right for you. When selecting
your type of yoga, think about what in particular makes you curious
about yoga. Is it the aspect of a new workout? A way to calm your
nerves? A new kind of stretch? Learning new poses in a fast-paced
way? Make note of which in this section align with your goals as a
budding yogi (or perhaps a well-seasoned yogi looking for something
to spice up your yoga life). Each style will bring something different
to the table.

VINYASA

❈ WHAT IS IT? The key to my heart is a wonderful Vinyasa flow. The strength you feel from taking your first chaturanga using your muscles to push you up and through is addicting (in a good way, of course). Vinyasa, simply, is the connection of breath and body. This particular type of yoga is the most mainstream and resonates with many. While some yoga practices are based on repetition, Vinyasa offers many different poses, so no two flows are the same. Using your breath to flow from one pose to another, you spend just enough time in each pose to find alignment, connect your breath, and then move on. Vinyasa flows mirror how we live life, in that everything is temporary. While some classes can be fast-paced, vigorous, challenging, and sweat-inducing, there are beginner Vinyasa yoga classes that can be softer, slow-flowing, gentle, and calming. Depending on the instructor, these classes can vary on pace and style.

❈ WHY DO IT? Fluidity. From my own personal practice, once I began to incorporate Vinyasa, my balance increased tremendously. The seamless transition from one pose evolving to another became easier, lighter, and less strenuous on my body. Along with this, there's something soothing about the methodical flow of a Vinyasa class. Wherever you are in your day, the ritual of starting class, going through poses in a sequenced flow, ending with a delicious savasana (mini nap session) while pumping your body with deep, luscious inhales, and exhaling the stress that you don't need is pure magic.

KUNDALINI

❀ WHAT IS IT? Kundalini yoga is a blend of Bhakti yoga, Raja yoga, and Shakti yoga (flip to chaper 4 for in-depth definitions of these types). Kundalini is energy coiled at the base of the spine. Conceptually, you're moving this energy from the spine through your chakras and to the brain, releasing it through chanting, dancing, and movement . . . which sounds like a party to me! It's a breathing party, if you will, as Kundalini brings insanely fierce breathwork into your life for long periods of time. Think less downdog, more breath of fire. Class ends with an extended savasana, which I must say, after a class of deep, deep, deep breathing, as well as poses and moves that require exceptional stamina and strength, is icing on a remarkable yoga-class cake.

❀ WHY DO IT? Talk about gland stimulus! Kundalini wakes everything up: the body, the breath, *everything*. It unlocks any tension you've been holding in, physically or mentally. The focus it requires to be present during class is fiery, requiring all the stamina you've got. Chanting may not be for everyone, and it takes a while to find the confidence to fully give over to making sounds in yoga, but combining all these efforts will make for an extremely unique yoga experience. During my training as an actor at a conservatory, one year we did yoga as a part of our curriculum. A year of Kundalini was so crucial to my progress, as it brought continual body awareness through intense breathwork. It was the perfect way to help me prepare for auditions; it required a different kind of commitment to myself that connected breath and body.

BIKRAM

❋ WHAT IS IT? Oh, Bikram, my love/hate relationship with yoga begins with you. Bikram is a ninety-minute yoga class in a sauna-like temperature. Repetition is an understatement when it comes to the twenty-six poses you do twice in a row in class, in the same order, with the same cues every. Single. Class. Bikram is not for the faint of heart, but rest assured, the feeling that you'll get after class is incomparable to any other sensation you've experienced. Your entire body post-class often feels completely flushed out: free of toxins—any drop of alcohol or fatty food you've consumed in the last month—leaving you feeling five pounds lighter and maybe a little light-headed. It is almost a euphoric state. I've found very few workouts or yoga classes that make me feel as refreshed as Bikram. But the process that leads to that result is a mental battle. You need to train yourself to not fidget between poses, to resist wiping sweat, fixing hair, and tugging at clothes. Training your mind and body to be present in this almost militarily precision is an adjustment, but it's well worth it.

❀ WHY DO IT? Every type of yoga is worth a try, and for anyone interested in yoga, I always suggest they try Bikram at some point. The requisite discipline alone is worth investigating, not only for your own practice, but for your everyday life. Bottom line: If you're looking for a good sweat and a feeling of body awareness for muscles you didn't even know existed, this class is for you.

HATHA

❀ WHAT IS IT? If you're looking for a slower-paced, uncomplicated, light introduction to yoga, Hatha is a safe place to begin. It encompasses all aspects of a generalized yoga class, so while you may not break a sweat, you will hold the positions a bit longer and work on refining each pose.

❀ WHY DO IT? I find Hatha to be extremely useful for balance as well as for increasing patience. On weeks when I'm feeling disconnected from my practice, I'll pop into a Hatha class for a reminder to slow down and reconnect with my muscles. It minimizes chance of injury, increases flexibility, and strengthens muscles, all while flexing the connection to body and mind. The pace of Vinyasa classes can sometimes be stressful, which cancels out the benefits of yoga for some people. So, for a less complicated experience, check out this style.

YIN

❈ **WHAT IS IT?** Yin yoga is specifically designed for slow muscle release. Based on the concept of yin and yang, these poses, which are very similar to Hatha, are designed to be practiced with less physical effort. There's major vulnerability when it comes to holding stretching poses for longer periods of time. While it can be physically freeing, Yin taps into the emotional side, too—allowing you to find meditation and relaxation throughout class. It requires focus and attention, as with Vinyasa or any other quick-paced class, so it's easy to assume what's next and jump ahead into the next pose. While a regular yoga practice is important, balancing out your stretching versus strength is just as necessary. Yin yoga allows you to physically and mentally deepen your practice.

❈ **WHY DO IT?** This class is perfect after one of those never-ending, stress-inducing days. While lubricating joints by spending extensive time in the poses and increasing mobility in the hips, it also brings focus to breathing through tougher poses. Personally, I feel the most tension in my body when I'm on the ground in restorative poses, as my body immediately goes into freak-out mode, saying, "Hey, wait! Your hips are tight—don't do that!" Yin will help guide your breath to parts of the body that need to find this release, all while increasing your ability to relax. There's an element of vulnerability when it comes to the lengthy time in these poses, which is an added element of challenge.

IYENGAR

❋ **WHAT IS IT?** Iyengar is really what brought the yoga we know today to the west, which makes it special. B. K. S. Iyengar, who founded this style of yoga, believed that to achieve a deeper sense of the pose, balance must be solid first. So in comparison to a Vinyasa flow, the poses are held longer and props are heavily encouraged. Iyengar's reach is holistic and extends to lifestyle habits. For example, in Iyengar's book, *Light on Yoga*, he specifically mentions how a yogi's eating habits correlate with practice, encouraging a well-maintained diet to help with your yoga. His process seriously highlights alignment in all aspects of life.

❋ **WHY DO IT?** If you're lacking understanding of alignment in your poses, Iyengar will refine your body awareness while continually sharpening your mind to proper positioning of yoga asanas. This yoga is for beginners or advanced yogis alike! One of the most important tools for your yogi tool belt is body awareness. Iyengar will bring your attention to muscles you didn't even know you had while building balance and increasing flexibility with the use of props. Lack patience? Iyengar will challenge you. It takes you beyond where you feel continually stuck, it teaches you about your body in small ways every class, and it shows you a different way to look at yoga, giving you nuggets of information to plug into your practice.

ASHTANGA

❀ **WHAT IS IT?** Similar to Vinyasa, Ashtanga is about quick-paced flow and linking breath and movement. It starts with ten rounds of sun salutations, poses on left and right sides, inversions, and, like Vinyasa, ends up with seated poses and stretching. If you're looking for a more in-depth, structured practice, Ashtanga is for you. As with Bikram, there is a very precise order of poses that you'll execute every class, so the repetition lends itself to quick and noticeable improvements in your strength, flexibility, and mental focus.

❀ **WHY DO IT?** When spicing up my yoga life, I tend to look for something that I typically would shy away from. I was always intimidated by the name Ashtanga, as I was unfamiliar with what it was exactly and only heard that it was difficult. Eventually I signed up for a class simply because it was the closest thing to me on a day where my body *really* needed a yoga class. Pleasantly surprised by how difficult it was, I realized that I sometimes judge a book by its cover when seeing unfamiliar names for yoga classes.

RESTORATIVE

❀ **WHAT IS IT?** Ah, Restorative yoga: The yoga class where you're encouraged to fall asleep. What a dream! In this class, you're asked to use extra props. Restorative yoga is a delicious treat of extended time in seated poses that are great for relieving stress, opening up, boosting your immune system, and quieting your mind. When dealing with emotional trauma or pain, restorative poses can help. They're also said to be useful for processing and handling depression, the loss of a loved one, the end of a relationship, or anything that's challenging you in the world of sadness. Restorative yoga helps in regrounding your mind and body. Essentially, this class is an hour for you to commit to alone time with yourself to just simply be and breathe.

❋ WHY DO IT? Restorative practice is for everyone, but especially those who have a hard time relaxing, meditating, or falling asleep (me!). One of my favorite memories was bouncing around the city working my three different jobs. I had an hour to kill in Manhattan and on a whim signed up for yoga. I didn't realize it was Restorative and initially was annoyed with myself for not double-checking, as I wanted to sweat and get a workout in. Upon arriving in class, I remember wanting it to be over already, my mind buzzing with all the tasks I had to do the rest of the day and frustrated that I had to just lie there in this Restorative class. I truly don't think I've ever experienced something so dreamy and refreshing. It was like someone pulled out every single negative thing that was weighing me down and tossed it out the window. I realized that my body was craving peace, groundedness, and extra breath more than a sweaty flow that day. The power of yoga is that it will heal you most if you allow yourself to listen to your body, and Restorative yoga is an excellent example of that.

ACRO

❀ **WHAT IS IT?** This is an alternative version of yoga. It may seem "too hard," or it may seem that you're not "good enough" to try it, but that's just not the case. If you've ever seen an Acro yoga class happening, you may have been amazed by the sight of people holding others up by their feet, spinning them around effortlessly and looking fabulous. Although Acro yoga can look complicated, here are the facts: You do not have to be a certain size to practice, and it's for everyone, even if you can't do any crazy acrobatics or even a handstand. There's a base, the yogi who supports most of the weight, similar to leg presses at the gym, who creates a sturdy foundation for play, and a flyer, who actively presses down with their weight as they're in the air being held by the base. With communication, trust, and abandonment of fear, you weight-share by creating a simultaneous push and pull with both bodies. It's definitely a more rigorous practice of yoga, but it still sticks to the philosophies, as well as the mental, physical, and spiritual aspects of other styles of yoga. It also incorporates aspects of Thai massage, if that sweetens the deal for you!

❀ **WHY DO IT?** If you're looking to meet new yogi friends, try something different and interesting, and build a strong core while improving your balance—all while up in the air—or if you want to do something different with a friend or partner, this is for you.

Remember, if you've been scared to give it a try, what's the harm in one class? You'll get some air time, a little bit of a massage, and a cool picture to show your friends that you were brave and tried something new.

AERIAL

❋ WHAT IS IT? Another alternative version of yoga, Aerial yoga, is where people are hanging upside-down from colorful silks! I've been teaching Aerial for going on three years and I must say, it's my all-time favorite. Aerial is the perfect way to deepen your yoga practice, and get some time upside-down. It takes traditional yoga poses and combines them with the Aerial hammock, which is fabric rigged from two points in the ceiling to create a U shape. It gives you the opportunity to refine poses without falling out and starting all over. There's also the element of going upside-down. I suffered a small lower back injury in college doing deadlifts (I've decided weight lifting is not for me), and my lifestyle in New York, characterized by sitting on the train too long, working seven- to ten-hour shifts as a front-desk receptionist, and walking everywhere, would cause me to wake up some mornings in excruciating pain. I began doing Aerial yoga regularly and quickly realized that I had eliminated pain around my sacrum through this practice. When inverting in your Aerial hammock, you're creating space in your vertebrae. After a few sessions of Aerial yoga, you can honestly feel like you're sitting taller. It's no illusion, just the magic of Aerial yoga!

❀ WHY DO IT? The most progress I've seen in any of my clients is through Aerial yoga, because we target core and arms. By working with the hammock as well as on the mat, you become very familiar with your body, both in mid-air and on the ground. Body awareness is a big part of this class, because there's an outside object you have to trust along with your own body. Plus . . . it is honestly so much fun. If you have lower back pain, GET YOURSELF INTO THIS CLASS. I swear by it.

POWER YOGA

❀ WHAT IS IT? Power yoga is a fitness-based Vinyasa flow, leaning hard into a modern-style yoga. I've seen a version of Power yoga at most bigger studios in New York City, and once I gave it a try I became addicted. Think (sometimes) hot yoga room, add some solid pump-up music and a faster flow, and you've got yourself a Power yoga class. It attracts the athletic crowd who like a spicy challenge while also getting their zen on. No chanting, less Sanskrit, more flow. This type of yoga can be seen in gym-type settings, and was created by Beryl Bender Birch and Bryan Kest to help introduce non-yogis to yoga. Power yoga will vary depending on teacher and location, so make sure to chat up your studio before giving it a try.

�֍ WHY DO IT? It's okay to want to do yoga for a workout! There isn't a yoga guru hiding behind the mirror making sure your yoga intentions are aligned. There are days I walk into class knowing that a hot Power yoga class is what my body needs to detox physically, and the mental part finds its way in naturally. When your body is properly engaged, you'll be sweating more than on a humid summer day in south Texas. Yoga has evolved in the same way we have as humans, and Power yoga is the perfect example of that. It allows you work with where you are to access your most true, full, and freest form and move in a way that is exhilarating and fulfilling.

❖ 4 ❖

WHAT'S THE BIG DEAL ABOUT YOGA?

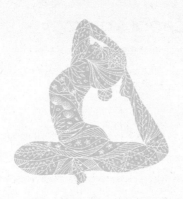

*"Yoga is not about touching your toes,
it's about what you learn on the way down."*

—JIGAR GOR

MUCH LIKE THE WAY CLASSES START WITH THE foundations, we've now gone over the basics of yoga. Let's add a layer to your understanding by answering the questions of what we're doing and why. We've got the body, we've got the breath, but why do we practice yoga? What makes yoga different than hopping into a workout class like cycling, kickboxing, barre, or pilates? You're moving your body, you're getting a physical workout . . . so what's the big deal about yoga?

This is where you can refine your practice and incorporate the philosophies that resonate most with you.

THE SIX SCHOOLS OF YOGA

Mainstream yoga generally refers to six separate "branches" of the tree of yoga: Bhakti, Karma, Jnana, Raja, Kriya, and Tantra.

Bhakti | Devote

As an instructor, Bhakti has been so important to my life, my personal practice, and how I move through each day. As an actor, judging myself and others was constantly at the forefront of my mind. While in audition rooms waiting for my time slot, I would immediately size up the competition, first analyzing if they'd get the part instead of me, then allowing self-doubt to take over my mind as I would begin to feel small, insecure, and unable to be the best version of myself. As I stepped into the shoes of being a yoga instructor, the judgmental veil was lifted. This part of me that was so deeply rooted through the world of acting began to fall away as I loved and welcomed every single person that walked into my classes. My acceptance of others through yoga has directly translated to how I interact with others on a daily basis. With Bhakti, you create room to cultivate acceptance of others. Bhakti is sacred. It's releasing, chanting, dancing, and moving.

Karma | Do

Karma is work—doing what you do with a spirit of selflessness. I feel like I'm a pretty decent human. Though I have flaws, I do my best to be kind, generous, a listener. But in my life there is a selfless person who's managed to completely change my perspective on what it means to truly give without expectation of receiving anything in return. We all have that one person in our lives whose light shines so bright, it is almost overwhelming (but in a good way). They speak badly of no one, encourage and uplift others during tough times without skipping a beat, and volunteer their time to others willingly, often and without asking a single thing in return. The way these types of people move through life inspires us to live without expectations of others, without needing a favor back in return—living simply and celebrating each day given to us. This directly translates to Karma yoga. Sri Sri Ravi Shankar once said, "When you make service your sole purpose in life, it eliminates fear, focuses your mind, and gives you meaning." Though we'd all like our sole purpose to be dedicated to others, obviously we can't get there overnight. Small random acts of kindness are a good start, as well as stepping back in the moments where you feel your ego taking over. When taking a yoga class, the teacher will occasionally offer you the option of dedicating your practice to someone. Even something small such as this can give energy back in a positive way.

Jnana | Discern

Some would say this is the trickiest path to master. The goal? To achieve harmony between one's self and all life. This is very reminiscent of those selfish desires we oh-so often shove to the backs of our minds. Jnana yoga is allowing yourself to let go of egotistical attitudes, or actions driven by desire. It's finding a way to maintain our true selves, controlling unwanted desires and centering ourselves to break free from the cycle of letting our ego take over. Jnana yoga is crucial in figuring out your own lessons and expressions of what life means to you. First, stabilize yourself. Second, find self-awareness. Third, combine self-awareness and awareness of what's around you. Fourth, add yoga.

Raja | Decide

Raja, also known as royal yoga, is heavily based on Patanjali's eight limbs of yoga (see page 37). Raja yoga is meditation plus contemplation, aka controlling thoughts with the practice of meditation. Moments when you can't focus before an interview, when you find yourself overly upset about something small, or when you're overly excited to the point of thinking about nothing else—this is where Raja comes in. When you master Raja, you gain the ability to tap in to a sense of balance and control of your emotions and mind. Raja brings your attention inward, assisting you in regulating your feelings toward a more simplistic way of living tied in with the eight limbs of yoga. Patanjali suggests simply sitting comfortably, focusing on breath and then mentally guiding your way through the limbs.

Kriya | Detox

Kriya yoga is the path of meditation, self-realization, and the ability to recognize the sorrow we bring upon ourselves through our actions. This one may sound intimidating. Few things are more terrifying than being alone with your thoughts for too long without being sure how to correctly "meditate." Kriya answers this fear by providing a path to flushing out bad thoughts and negative vibes, burning away anything you don't need. We work with the deep spiritual energies intertwined with our spine by turning attention to breath.

Tantra | Dance

This yoga form is all about the body, bringing about both strength and vulnerability in yourself. I suppose many people would aquaint Tantra yoga with sex as well, but it's much more than that. Pushing forth confidence within yourself, Tantra yoga encourages connecting energies within yourself to others and the universe. So yes, if you're looking to find a deeper connection with your partner and want to explore something beyond physical intimacy, with Tantra you're in the right place. Tantric yoga is meant to refine your emotional life and tap in to your physical connection, even though it's most known for sexual empowerment through healing with yoga, or known as a way to connect with your partner sexually through Tantra yoga. In my 200hr, the most basic and necessary yoga certification, we focused on Tantra as modifying—in other words, refining and listening to when your body isn't ready for a certain pose or needs a break. Tantra is listening to your body when it tells you something isn't right, but it's also gaining the ability to stay with sensations that your body is uncomfortable with—not excruciating pain or something that is harming the body, but maybe something you avoid because of insecurity. My favorite phrase passed down from my teacher and mentor Courtney Bauer, founder of Studio ANYA, is "Modification is a sign of wisdom." This phrase opens the door many of my clients are looking for to take their first steps into a safe and welcoming practice. It allows their bodies and minds to feel at home when stepping onto their mat, to honor how their bodies are feeling. Finding that connection is so important. There are many elements to Tantra, many workshops created for anyone looking to take their sexual life beyond just a physical sensation. Tantra can help to connect with intimacy, the heart chakra, or in finding a deeper relation with your significant other, or it can be a way of connecting emotionally with yourself.

WHY ARE THESE IMPORTANT TO YOUR PRACTICE?

I like to think of yoga as a big layered cake. Sure, the first layer of poses is fine. You can eat a tiny piece of it and you're satisfied. But, adding another layer—breath—makes it even tastier, as well as visually satisfying.

What about a third layer? That's kind of what the branches of yoga are. They add the fullness to the cake, rounding out your experience of enjoying every last bite. The branches of yoga add purpose, guidance, and deliciousness to your practice.

Most seek yoga as a way of becoming more flexible, as a different approach to fitness, or maybe because a doctor recommended it as a way to ease back into movement after an injury. Once you're in class, you'll start to realize it's so much more than just physically challenging: it's mentally challenging you to seek your inner truth. It's satisfying to align your body with your mind, your goals, what you want out of life. Sometimes it takes you by surprise. There are days when I've gone to class just to move a little and I come out on the other side feeling like all my life problems have been addressed because of the dharma talk (the little speech you hear from some yoga instructors if you start or end class in meditation), which is that last bit of icing on the cake. It adds an element of depth to movement. Everyone in the room around you is experiencing the same thing, and, as a collective, you're rooting yourself in something beautiful while simultaneously interpreting it in your own, intimate way.

❖ 5 ❖

THE
EIGHT
LIMBS

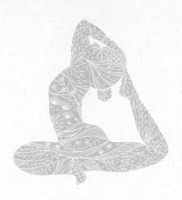

"Yoga is the journey of the self, through the self, to the self."

—BHAGAVAD GITA

INALLY, ONCE YOU'VE BECOME FAMILIAR WITH the different schools and philosophies, you can begin to study the famous eight limbs of yoga. As you begin your physical practice, this can be layered on over time. There's no need for you to feel like a super yogi, mastering a meaningful and fulfilled life right away and all at once. Even with years of practice under my belt, there are certain limbs that are harder for me to integrate into my life and practice than others. The eight limbs of yoga have added so much to my life, as well as the way I teach my classes. There's a moral concept to each one, which helps guide you toward bettering your health and mind.

FIRST LIMB:
YAMA—UNIVERSAL MORALITY

The first part, yama, is ourselves in relation to the outside world. How our actions affect us, as well as the people we interact with, and the world at large.

1. Ahimsa—Nonviolence, Compassion for All Living Things

We all know violence is never the answer. But, as obvious as that statement can be, I like to think of violence in a less physical sense, but rather in the small, seemingly insignificant thoughts that consume us throughout the day. Ahimsa is the act of refraining from not only physical violence, but emotional and mental violence as well.

❀ **HOW TO PRACTICE IT EVERY DAY:** If I enjoy a cheesy slice of pizza, then turn around and spend the rest of the day obsessing over how guilty I feel that I indulged in a craving, I'm creating mental violence. Forgiving yourself for something you've done, or doing the same for others in your life, is a way of practicing nonviolence. High expectations of yourself or others is another version of violence. The most important thing you can do for yourself to incorporate ahimsa into your life is to accept things as they are while letting go of your expectations. Once, while grabbing coffee at a local shop, I forgot cash and the man behind me offered to pay for my coffee. If I were to expect someone to pay for my coffee *every* time I went to the coffee shop, that would make me look and feel insane. Expectations of people and yourself create complications if they aren't fulfilled as planned. It goes the same way for holding on to things that create mental and physical tension. When you resent others, you are cultivating negativity for yourself and everyone around you. Changing the way we think is, of course, easier said than done; but the more we let life happen rather than force friendships, relationships, and situations, the more at peace our minds and bodies feel.

❀ ON THE MAT: By practicing yoga, you're calming the mind, the body, and the spirit. Letting go of any negative thoughts that have clouded your mind that day invites a clean slate for positivity.

2. Satya—Truthfulness, Commitment to Honesty

Satya is truthfulness in our thoughts and speech—another yama that's easier said than done. We all strive to be honest and truthful, but no one is perfect! Satya means fighting against the pattern of overbooking schedules, making promises to friends, family, and work, but, when the time comes, realizing you have no energy left for yourself.

❀ HOW TO PRACTICE IT EVERY DAY: Practicing self-care is crucial to truthfulness, because it means that you're being honest to both yourself and others about how much you can or can't do. When you have obligations but you know that you've overcommitted, simply saying, "I need to take some time for myself tonight. Thank you for the invite, and I'll catch you sometime next week" instead of making up an excuse opens your heart to being honest with yourself and friends. White lies are easy, but in a way it's like putting a Band-Aid on a broken bone. You have done nothing to fix the situation, and may have even made it worse by ignoring the issue upfront. The pain of the truth will sting sharply at first, but will be far less painful than a white lie that resurfaces weeks or months later.

❀ ON THE MAT: During yoga, the truthfulness of honoring your body and mind during class is a way of bringing satya into your practice. If you're feeling pain in your wrists, popping up into a handstand during class is a major disservice to your body and likely will result in a painful and potentially dangerous outcome. Taking a moment to acknowledge where you're at that day is being honest with where you are in your practice.

3. Asteya—Non-stealing

Why do people steal? What is the root of something so nasty and greedy? I think back to when I was in school for theater, and comparison surfaced almost constantly. In my head, I would belittle others in order to give myself confidence: I took something away from a person that made them who they were in order to give myself something that I lacked. I always felt like there was a part of myself that was unsettled or unsatisfied with my looks or my talents. When we feel as though we lack something, the needy-greedy side kicks in. That little voice we talked about earlier, the "I'm not good enough," or the "they're better than me" is a way of stealing from yourself and stealing from others. Another form of asteya is robbing yourself and others of an experience for selfish reasons. We see this often in children, where they're completely unaware of how their actions when they're upset affect those around them. A small temper tantrum could ruin any kind of gathering. As an adult, I commonly see this when insecurities are present. To make themselves feel comfortable, they will shut down or reject an event or experience to create a comfortable space, not realizing how it could negatively affect those attempting to enjoy what's around them.

❁ **HOW TO PRACTICE IT EVERY DAY:** Don't be that person who comes in five minutes late, whispering you're sorry while flopping your mat awkwardly down hoping someone will make space for you. This is stealing! You're taking away someone's experience of yoga by disrupting their class. I get it, traffic is bad some days, you forgot something and had to go back home, you don't want to lose the money that you paid for the class or not get your practice in; but by arriving late you've robbed others *and* yourself. Along with this, yoga's literal definition is "yoke" or "unity," which means whole. By coming to class, you are bringing together your mind, body, and spirit to make the whole. Finding your inner source of happiness will keep you from reaching outward for a sense of wholeness.

❋ ON THE MAT: While in class, do your best to be as present as possible with yourself. As soon as you begin to occasionally steal glances at your neighbor, trying to mimic what they're doing instead of intuitively listening to what your body's telling you, your class has been stolen and replaced with a completely different experience. Once those thoughts of "I want to do what they're doing" or "well, they're clearly doing this better" begin to take over, you've robbed yourself of a successful class.

4. Brahmacharya—Continence, Sense Control

This, admittedly, isn't the most popular of the yamas—its literal translation is "celibacy" or "to be celibate." The classical definition of this term refers to refraining from sexual desires to gain strength, and your sexual energy to be directed toward your yoga practice as opposed to the act of sex itself. But hold on, before you skip this section, give it a chance. I read once that the more obsessed you are with something, the more you lose control. By abstaining, you're able to find strength, rather than being controlled by these desires. So look at this yama in a less literal sense: The things we lust after may be distracting us from what will actually give us true happiness and peace.

❋ HOW TO PRACTICE IT EVERY DAY: Let's chat about how to make brahmacharya a realistic goal. On days where you use the excuse "I'm just too busy," what are you actually doing? Where are you dedicating your energy? If you're filling your days with activities to seem successful, or filling your time with people who aren't contributing to your overall betterment, this energy is being wasted. Learning to say no to projects that don't drive your passion can be a big deal. For example, I spent a lot of my first few years in the city doing work that drained my soul. On the outside, I kept telling myself that I was successful because my schedule was full and I was doing what I loved. Looking deeper, the projects I was committing my time to had sucked the energy out of me and I felt like I had to say yes to every friend, every project, every job. I now direct my energy toward people who inspire me, who support me just as much as I support them, and projects that spark interest and light a fire in my work ethic. Brahmacharya encourages your energy to be used positively, so take a few moments in your day when feeling overly busy to take some deep yoga breaths, ask yourself "Will this matter a year from now?" and proceed with your day. Allow yourself to take control of what your days are made up of.

✤ ON THE MAT: When first doing Bikram, I used to obsess over certain poses. I would get overly excited in class whenever it was time to come into those poses, and every single bit of my energy would be poured into those couple of moves. When it came time to move forward, I was physically exhausted, which resulted in my continually (Every. Single. Class. for six years . . .) skipping the same two poses that I hated. As a result, my class was completely uneven. If you're in class and find your mind wandering to "I dislike how I look in this pose" or "I'm not good enough to do this pose," focus on breathing through the mind chatter and spending the same amount of confidence, perseverance, and energy for every single pose. It gives you that control over not obsessively hating or loving any particular poses, but truly spending your energy evenly.

5. Aparigraha—Non-possessiveness; Take What Is Necessary

Learning how to let that sh*t go is one of the hardest yamas to incorporate into life, on the mat and beyond. As you go through life, the sooner you realize you must let go of things you don't need in order to move forward, there will be a new sense of peace in existing. This will resonate with you if you're in a spot where letting go is challenging. In your yoga practice, if you continually hold on to that one class where you nailed every pose, did the best warrior 3 of your life, and felt like you were on cloud nine after, you'll have an extremely tough yoga path. Right before the final savasana, I tell my class to take a moment of gratitude for coming to class today, for moving as their body allowed them to move on that day, in that hour with the breath that arrived. I then ask them to exhale that day's practice away, forever cleaning the slate for the next time. You must allow experiences to be with you in a way that is not obsessive, or keeps you from moving to the next thing. Similarly, we shouldn't cling to good things either, since we will close ourselves off from potential new good things.

✤ **HOW TO PRACTICE IT EVERY DAY:** I find this yama to be especially necessary to how we live in the modern day. We are presented with so many physical objects, friendships, and ideas of what we want and need that it clouds who we are. Attaching yourself to one person so much that you lose yourself is dangerous as well. My favorite way of seeing a relationship isn't "we complete each other" or "they're my other half," but you are already whole to begin with, and the other person is just bringing out the best parts of you. Do your best to live in the present as much as possible. Let go of the parts of your past that no longer serve you, and don't attach yourself to certain life paths, allowing space between you and what's to come. The best way to practice aparigraha is to forgive and forget. Let go of resentment, whether it be a fight with a friend, an awful day at work, a string of negative things that leads to one right after another, or anything that keeps you from a clearer mind.

✤ **ON THE MAT:** Find your breath, and let that be your guide to exhaling the things weighing you down. As you go through each yoga class, the more focused your breath is on continually cleaning your slate and staying in the room, the better you'll feel post-class. If I lived in the past of every yoga class I've ever taken, I would never make any progress physically or mentally. It would be silly to hear someone say, "Two years ago in one particular yoga class, my tree pose was the best ever." I'm positive even my yoga pals would furrow their brows and look at me in confusion if I were to talk like that. The whole point of coming to class is to make progress, and if you're mentally holding on to the one time you think you nailed class and did so great, you're keeping yourself from having one hundred classes that were equally as great.

SECOND LIMB: NIYAMA—OBSERVATION OF SELF

Turning the mirror back on yourself can be the hardest part about venturing into the yoga world. I noticed a big shift in the way I lived life once I started actually listening to my dharma before class. I began to practice what I preach, attempting to reach my own personal, inner truth. On days when I feel in over my head, I take a moment to mentally step aside and look at how far I've come. Take your time with niyamas. When allowing yourself to crack open this part of your soul, be kind, be self-aware, and cultivate a positive and loving relationship with you.

1. Sauca—Cleanliness

The feeling of making your bed before you leave for the day is so satisfying, why not do it more? A clean physical space leads to a clear mind. I spent many days in college avoiding work simply because my room wasn't organized. Somehow, tossing my laundry in the hamper, putting all my desk trinkets in their places, and emptying the trash made my mind at ease to memorize my Shakespeare for class, or finish my text analysis for a scene I was doing in acting class. Physically clearing your space makes way for your mind to settle into what needs to get done, or even to do something as simple as fall asleep at night. While practicing yoga, keeping your focus in the room, on yourself, with your breath is a way of including sauca in your yoga world.

❀ HOW TO PRACTICE IT EVERY DAY: Mentally, we strive for cleanliness. Get rid of jealousy, greed, and negativity. The last time you were really, really angry or upset, did you feel it physically? Maybe your shoulders were up to your ears, jaw clenched, fists balled up, nails digging into your skin. Something as simple as a giant exhale can free your body from the built-up tension a cluttered mind accumulates. A clearer mind leads to less aggression in our muscles. This doesn't mean you should deny your feelings. But let these feelings be visitors only. When they begin to inhabit your mind, you suffer physically and emotionally. In acting classes, students are asked to think of a story from their lives that carries with it a physical feeling. Recounting that experience might produce a pain in the gut, a tingly feeling in the heart, a sharpness in the chest, a warm sensation in the belly. This illustrates how deeply our thoughts and experiences live in our bodies. If we practice sauca, we free ourselves from the pain of these sensations and can think more objectively about our needs.

❀ ON THE MAT: While practicing yoga, keeping your focus in the room and on yourself with your breath is a way of including sauca in your yoga world. Do your best to leave any clutter outside the room. Put the mind chatter on pause as you cleanse your thoughts, your mat, and your space in preparation for a focused and well-balanced class. Wipe away any unnecessary stress that won't serve you for the hour you'll be yogaing.

2. Samtosa—Contentment, Inner Satisfaction

The niyamas guide us to better relationships with ourselves. Samtosa is defined as inner satisfaction, being content with what's in front of you. Not to say we shouldn't set goals, have standards for living, or aspire to be the best we can be. But samtosa means finding moments of gratitude in the little things we have right in front of us.

❋ HOW TO PRACTICE IT EVERY DAY: It can be hard not to battle samtosa on a daily basis, immediately jumping to the next thing once you've checked an item off your to-do list. To slow down, you might consider daily gratitudes. At the end of each day, name three things you're grateful for, whether it be coffee in the morning or a new job opportunity. Even if you're living a life you love, it's possible to feel somewhat unsatisfied. In those moments, it's okay to take a step back and think "Look at how far I've come!" with a breath of relief. We bury our heads in our work so much at times, we forget to look back at all we've accomplished to get to where we are. If we're working toward a goal for our whole life without an ounce of satisfaction throughout the journey, what's the point?

❁ ON THE MAT: It's easy to break that focus as your gaze drifts toward the yogi next to you, shattering the small amount of samtosa you'd gathered in your practice. You were fine with how your dancer pose looked, you felt confident and content with today's practice, and then BOOM. That little bit of doubt that it could maybe be better led you outside of yourself and into the battle of your inner self not being satisfied. Appreciate your body and how far you've come with every class. There may be times when life leads you away from your mat due to physical injury, emotional trauma, or whatever it may be. Know that your practice is something that will never leave you, but that it will change and fluctuate over time. The quicker you can value yourself and find peace with where you are, the deeper your practice will be.

3. Tapas—Energy, Heat

Rooting from the Sanskrit word *tap*, which translates to *burn* as in *to burn away*, or *to evoke passion*, tapas can be seen for the actual sense of creating heat on the mat, or the idea of "burning away" what you don't need.

❁ HOW TO PRACTICE IT EVERY DAY: What's the best way to burn off the negativity? Maybe it's drinking extra water before bed to ensure a well-hydrated yoga practice the next day, grabbing a salad instead of nachos after class to put good fuel in your body, or even taking a few moments before a stressful day to be with your breath, meditating.

There's a big difference between pushing yourself when your body says no, and what the discipline of tapas is. The uplifting encouragement of finding just how long you can hold that crow pose or using your breath to fuel you through poses can come in handy off your mat when getting through a stressful situation. When I get jitters before an audition, my hands get really sweaty, my legs feel heavy, and I feel as though I've swallowed a rock. I begin to doubt my abilities, think of horrible ways I can possibly mess up the audition, begin to wonder if I still have the words memorized, and slowly begin to spiral to a very negative place. When this kicks in, my go-to tapas is "breath of fire" (see page 56). It calms me immediately, and is almost like hitting a hard reset. My body recognizes it as a way to cool off, calm down, and let go of the negative scenario I created for myself.

❀ ON THE MAT: On days when we have no desire to practice, tapas knocks on the door to entice us to the mat. Or perhaps it's that slight bit of encouragement we need to stay in that crow pose five seconds longer despite the want to give up. Tapas will be different for you than others; it's your form of discipline. How to tap into *tap*as? Find what ignites and inspires you. If you want to do yoga to start your day, go to bed earlier. Get tired toward the end of yoga practice? Eat a little something before you start. The key to successfully finding this passionate energy is to identify what's lacking or what is keeping you from finding that edge in your practice and in your life.

4. Svadhyaya—Scriptures/Self-study

Svadhyaya is translated directly to self-study. We're starting to wade pretty deep into the limbs of yoga, and this one in particular can take your practice beyond the mat and into your life. It encourages us to look at habits, thought process, and actions and figure out the root of why we do what we do. The meaning of yoga is to unite, to bring you closer to your true self. Svadhyaya begins to knit that together by assessing small intentional or unintentional doings that have pulled us further away from where we are truly rooted.

❀ **HOW TO PRACTICE IT EVERY DAY:** The scriptural aspect of understanding the yamas and niyamas doesn't mean you have to crack open the Bhagavad Gita and begin memorizing every inspiring phrase. Even reading this book is a way of bringing svadhyaya into daily use. But, if you read a thousand articles, books, and yoga magazines it wouldn't matter if it's not absorbed correctly. It's the understanding of the "scriptures" in relation to your own life that correlates with svadhyaya. Basically, it's like studying for any kind of daily quiz like the ones you had in high school. If you did the bare minimum to get the material in your head without honestly digesting any real information, you won't remember anything after taking the test. Find yoga material that excites you, ignites you, and taps into what resonates with your soul.

Observing behavior can be scary, and the realization of behavior once brought to life can be even scarier. I spent six years in a relationship with someone who made me unhappy for the last two legs of it; but because of the time spent with this person, I habitually ignored warning signs of emotional trauma. Even though things were horrible, I remember thinking, "Well, it could be worse." I had a tipping point, a moment where it became clear just how much of myself I was sacrificing for someone who wasn't right for me. I got to this point by observing my behavior when friends would try to talk to me about why I was still with him. I noticed how defensive my body would get, how I refused to make eye contact, how I felt a gnawing pain in my gut as if I was lying anytime I said I was happy. There it was, right in front of my face, the shattering reality that I'd drifted so far from my true self, my wants, desires, hopes, dreams, all the tiny things that pieced together to form *me*. Like Dorothy collecting the Scarecrow, Tin Man, and Lion, I scraped up the parts of me that had been lost for a while and took steps closer to uniting my true being. I still think back to that time and wonder how it got to the point of being so blind to what was right in front of me.

We all do it, in small ways. Maybe when someone compliments you, your first reaction is to reject nice words because it's hard for you to see what they see. Maybe you tell little white lies to spare feelings. Observe your reactions to a shift in plans, when someone doesn't get back to you immediately, when it rains unexpectedly, when you fall out of warrior 3, when downdog is more difficult than usual. You have so many secrets within you that will tell you how to tap into your true self—are you willing to find out the answers?

❁ **ON THE MAT:** It's easy to be distracted by mirrors or the people around you, but when you focus 100 percent of your attention on YOU, your ego is pushed aside and you're able to notice small habits in your practice that have been keeping you from moving forward. For example, those six years I spent avoiding triangle in Bikram because I was always "too tired." (I wasn't too tired; I was just afraid it looked bad.)

Noticing the way your body reacts to certain poses, where your mind goes for each asana or how your body reacts to uncomfortable positions may directly reveal how you handle similar situations in life. Do you skip and back out instead of confronting issues head-on? Your mat life is way more intertwined into your real life than you think.

5. Isvara Pranidhana—Spiritual Celebration

Something that I feel is important to say especially when talking about yoga is that your spiritual celebration is *yours*. There are some yogis who are strict in their beliefs of religion in relation to yoga, but this doesn't mean YOU have to agree with it. Take what you're taught with a grain of salt, but allow yourself to surrender to the practice fully. Isvara pranidhana is the act of surrendering—to a higher power, to something out there bigger than yourself. If *god* is a scary word that doesn't strike you in a comfortable way, think of this in terms of "letting go." We feel the need to meticulously control every single part of our lives that we forget that no matter how badly we want something, sometimes it won't happen. Maybe it will happen at a later point, or even in a different way than we wanted. If a "higher power" isn't what floats your boat, try just simply surrendering control.

❀ HOW TO PRACTICE IT EVERY DAY: Think about the last time you really enjoyed a meal. You tasted every last morsel and had full appreciation for each bite. You felt satisfied afterward. Or when was the last time you enjoyed a friend's company without looking at your phone? Surrendering to the moment fully, taking it into your mind, heart, and body to its full extent and being present is isvara pranidhana in real life.

❀ ON THE MAT: Surrender to the uncomfortableness of a position. In that moment in dancer when you typically fall out because it's hard, push past that and linger in the pose ten seconds longer. Surrender to actually *being* in the pose, feeling the breath and stability you've created.

Yay, we did it! Now that you've been introduced to the yamas and niyamas, may your practice be guided by these very quick summaries of their lessons.

THIRD LIMB:
ASANA—PHYSICAL POSES

Don't you worry, we've got a whole chapter dedicated to this. See page 73 for more.

FOURTH LIMB:
PRANAYAMA—BREATH CONTROL

Welcome to one of the most important parts of yoga: breathing! I heard once that at the bottom of our exhale we feel most like ourselves. In that moment, we are our best versions of who we are. Think about it: When you get the phone call you've waited for all week, when the train comes right within your window of being on time, when you receive good news, they all are usually followed with a giant sigh of relief, and we feel back to normal again. When you have a stressful day, you're about eight seconds away from feeling 50 percent better. Four-second breath in, exhale, four-second breath out. You've set a reset button to sustain you throughout the day, to keep you moving forward when it feels like you're at a loss. Pranayama means "to extend vital life force" so essentially, taking five minutes a day to center your breath will be giving you back your life and is incredibly important in creating balance within yourself.

Different Types of Breath

Going back to the Vedas, there are around fifty different types of breathing. I've pulled together some of the most popular types that are accessible to any and all.

BREATH AWARENESS

❊ HOW TO DO IT: Start by lying on your back, with palms to the sky and full body relaxed. Start to notice the physical sensation of when your rib cage expands and your lower belly empties. Take one hand to your heart, one hand to your lower belly. Use this tactile feedback to observe your breath. Where are you holding tension, even in the most relaxed pose you could be in? Is there unevenness in your breath cycles? Begin to take deep breaths in and out for six to twelve cycles.

❊ WHY DO IT? With all we have going on as humans, breath is the last thing on our minds. So what happens to your body when you lie down and actually turn your attention to your ribcage? This helps bring awareness to your breath and body, as well as create a sense of calmness in your mind. You might find it useful to go through this process on nights when you have difficulty sleeping.

BREATH OF FIRE

❊ HOW TO DO IT: Make your spine tall, but sit comfortably. Start with a natural breath, noticing your inhale and exhale. Begin to pump the stomach from the navel with your inhale and exhale. Keep your mouth open as you begin as if you're panting like a dog. Close your mouth and find the breath just through the nose. Quicken your pace while keeping your inhale and exhale the same length. Start with one to three rounds, then eventually work in five to ten. Breath of fire is purifying your oxygen.

✾ WHY DO IT? As I mentioned earlier, this is my go-to breath when I'm nervous or have a lot of extra energy that isn't serving me. It regulates my breath while calming my mind. Afterward, I feel like I've put that buzzing energy to good use instead of it making me nervous. Breath of fire also strengthens the core while activated. Who knew breath could be a way of trimming the belly? It's invigorating, meditative, and will leave you feeling slightly light-headed in a way that makes your skull feel warm and hugged.

DO NOT DO THIS if you're pregnant or have vertigo,
high blood pressure, or abdominal pain.

UJJAYI BREATH

✾ HOW TO DO IT: Find a comfortable seat. Place your palms on top of your thighs. Begin your natural breath. As you exhale through the mouth, make an *ahhh* sound (like waves in an ocean or like you're heating up your throat). Once your breath is regulated, same as with breath of fire, close your mouth. Breathe only through your nose. You should feel the same "ahhh" sensation in your throat as when the mouth was open. Let the sound of your breath relax you. Start for a few minutes, eventually expanding your time to fifteen minutes of Ujjayi breath. Steadiness is important, so if you feel out of control during your breath cycles, slow it down even more.

❋ WHY DO IT? This breath might be familiar to you, as I've experienced it in many Vinyasa flows, as well as Bikram. Ujjayi translates to "to conquer" or "to be victorious," which makes sense, since it can produce a feeling of empowerment as you take over your own breath. I've heard it referred to as "ocean's breath" as well because of how it sounds. It can be taxing on the throat after a while, and takes getting used to, but it has many benefits besides making you sound like a badass. Often, teachers will use this breath for a lengthy yoga class. Ujjayi breath does just that while keeping you grounded and is useful for headaches.

LION'S BREATH

❋ HOW TO DO IT: Sit on your heels. Place your hands on your knees with arms extended. Inhale through the nose. Exhale, making a "ha" sound while sticking your tongue out as far as you can (roaring like a lion!). Set your gaze to your third eye (aka cross your eyes—don't be afraid to look silly!). Inhale to neutral face. Repeat four to seven times.

❋ WHY DO IT? Lion's breath is a good reminder not to take yourself so seriously. It's also said to rid the body of disease, stimulate platysma (muscle in the neck), and help get rid of bad breath. It warms up the muscles in the face while opening the throat chakra, much like Ujjayi warms up the body as well.

DIRGA

❧ **HOW TO DO IT:** Lie on your back with either legs extended or feet flat with the knees resting on each other. Beginning to layer your breath, start with a simple inhale and exhale. Start to deepen your breath cycles, expanding your belly like blowing up a balloon. Adding in part two, fill your belly to the maximum, to just where you don't think you can sip in more air, expanding the rib cage and belly. To exhale, reverse how you began by letting the air seep out from the ribs, then the belly. Repeat this a few times. Inhale belly fully, inhale ribs, and then one final inhale to the heart space and collarbones. For the exhalation, start with your heart, then empty from your ribs, then empty from the balloon belly.

❧ **WHY DO IT?** I find Dirga to be the most calming of all pranayama breathing that I've experienced. Ending class with the ritual three-part breath is soothing to the mind and body, helping my students drift into savasana. I'll often cue a normal breath in and out, inhale one third into the lower belly, inhale up into the rib space, inhale up into the heart space, exhale the biggest sigh you've found all class, then repeat five times, allowing them the freedom to carry it with them into their final rest or to come back to the normal breath.

When you increase your oxygen, you decrease stress and anxiety. I would also suggest finding time in your day for five minutes of Dirga. Now, the next time your coworker is giving you major anxiety, it's not wise to drop onto your back and start Dirga for fear of confusing your office . . . but if you happen to feel major uneasiness in your chest, this is your go-to move. There are no crazy throat-breathing or sounds that need to be made, just being aware of your body and breath.

BHRAHAMARI

❀ HOW TO DO IT: Find a comfortable seat. Shut your eyes and begin to take deep breaths. Gently close your ears by plugging them with your thumbs. Place your index fingers above your eyebrows and the rest of your fingers on your eyelids. Apply gentle pressure to the sides of the nose. Keep your mouth closed as you breathe out the sound of *om*. During this process, you are connecting to the positive energies the universe has to offer.

❀ WHY DO IT? *Bzzzzzzz*—this is known as the "bee breath" because of how it sounds! Bhrahamari relaxes the mind, reduces stress, and has been said to cure paralysis and migraines. With the eyes and ears closed, the buzzing activates and awakens a sense of seclusion. Whenever I do Bhrahamari breathing, I feel like I'm able to escape to a secluded place miles away from the world for a few brief moments to reduce stress or calm my brain. One fact that struck me about Bhrahamari breathing is that it dissipates anger. I have been trying it out anytime I've found myself feeling extremely frustrated. I'll take five to ten rounds at a time, and I can say it slows my inner tempo down, as if I'm wrapping myself into my own little blanket of buzzing. The next time you go to dig into your leftover pizza and you find your roommate finished it off, take to Bhrahamari first before sending that angry text.

FIFTH LIMB: PRATYAHARA—CONTROL OF SENSES

This limb is associated with savasana, the lying-down pose normally done at the end of a yoga class, and translates to "the conscious withdrawal of energy from the senses." Though it can be lovely and cozy, the first part of savasana is only the beginning of controlling your senses. There are moments in savasana when you're not quite asleep, but it feels like everything is far away from you. Perhaps you've reached a state where thoughts about everything outside of the room have dissipated, and while you're aware, you're still *you* in your body in this room, but have no response to outside stimulus. This is pratyahara. You've shed your layers and have tapped into a sense of withdrawing from your mental "sheath." According to yoga philosophy, we all have five sheaths:

1. THE FOOD SHEATH, WHICH IS THE PHYSICAL BODY: our bones, organs, etc.

2. **THE PRANA SHEATH, THE ENERGY BODY, IS WHAT KEEPS US GOING, OUR VITALS:** the force and drive behind your cells, atoms, etc., and the systems that control taking in air and getting rid of waste.

3. **THE MENTAL SHEATH, MIND/BODY/NERVOUS SYSTEM:** your feelings, how you process the outside world and what's around you; you absorb everything through your senses, which are included in the mental sheath.

4. **THE CONSCIOUSNESS SHEATH, THE WISDOM BODY:** This is your gut feeling, working on developing your connection with yourself to fine-tune that awareness. Choosing when to let your consciousness sheath guide you becomes crucial to how you live your life.

5. **THE BLISS SHEATH:** Exactly how the name is understood, this is your true moment of peace—the first warm day of spring, sipping coffee on a rainy day, smelling roses, honey, watching a good movie, losing yourself fully in something that brings joy to your senses.

Our inner peace is precious, and though our world can be exciting and amazing, there are elements that add stress. I think about it like Alice in Wonderland when she starts to fall down the rabbit hole. We see Alice falling, unable to grasp what's around her, suspended in a moment where she's unattached to her world above, but there's a sense of euphoria about the distance between her and her physical self. Pratyahara isn't about hiding from the world and secluding yourself from the sheaths that make up who you are, it's about being able to find a moment of neutrality and peace without losing your senses. When you're able to shed these layers, you have withdrawn these senses and made yourself available for pratyahara.

❀ HOW TO PRACTICE IT EVERY DAY: With social media, I wake up and am informed about fifteen different awful things that have happened overnight around the world within the span of five minutes. Immediately, I want to shut down. I feel like I've taken on the weight of these terrible things, even though none may directly connect with my life. We are not meant to take this burden with us throughout the day. In the same realm, even positive social media can be just as taxing. We all have moments of scrolling through social media seeing friends doing only fun things, models, advertisements, and seemingly perfect lives popping up one after another. Begin by eliminating as much negative content as you can, when you can. Don't read that article with the graphic photo attached, unfollow that picture-perfect blogger who makes you feel like you're not good enough, remove toxic people in your life or friends who no longer support or uplift you, or those who talk negatively or aggressively.

The second thing you can do to bring more pratyahara into your life is to surround yourself with things that bring your soul joy. I love buying myself flowers and keeping them in rooms I spend a lot of time in. The littlest things can uplift our senses. Reconnect with nature. Consider finding a temporary escape from your everyday life and taking a short trip to the beach, the mountains, or another area where you can disconnect and recharge. Sit on the beach with your toes in the sand and sun on your skin while the waves crash—being in nature can be a total cleanse for your senses. You'll feel refreshed and ready to take on the world. Eat veggies, drink water, burn candles, get a diffuser and load it up with lavender scents—do all the things you tell yourself you'll eventually do but end up forgetting. Take control of your senses and feed them with rich, beautiful stimulants to carry the burden of what's bad in this world. It's not about running away or ignoring our problems, but being present and choosing to be positive, to find peace, to remove what no longer serves you. The more care you put into your life, the deeper your meditation will be.

❀ON YOUR MAT: Be present; focus on your breath. When outside elements start to worm their way into your mind throughout your practice, let them go and move forward. During savasana, remember that whatever is happening after class, outside the room, later that week—that will all still be there after you take this moment for yourself.

SIXTH LIMB:
DHARANA—INNER AWARENESS

The last three limbs are typically strung together like a bow on a wrapped present. As a yoga instructor who's also established a career in acting and photography, dharana is particularly difficult for me to fully embrace. The ability to fully submerge yourself in one thing—running five miles, singing through the entire *Hamilton* Broadway recording, finishing a piece of art you've been working on, keeping your mind totally focused on one activity for a length of time—is HARD. When this singular focus is achieved, you'll feel blissful and calm. Committing all of your concentration to each of your passions all at once is an impossible proposition—dharana is the ability to quiet the mind and turn your attention to one specific thing.

❀ HOW TO PRACTICE IT EVERY DAY: Think about when you wake up and reach for your phone. How many different apps do you check before getting out of bed? From one to another, you bounce back and forth. While eating breakfast, you maybe multitask by reading the paper or latest article that's popped up on your newsfeed. If you're reading a book, how much of it are you digesting and how much of your mind has started to get distracted, leading you to text a friend? When meeting someone new, how quickly do you forget their name because you weren't actually listening for it and instead were just focused on yourself? Dharana can't be achieved if you spread your attention span too thin. While in yoga class, can you commit your mind 100 percent to the task in front of you? Can you fully give yourself over to the poses and the breath?

✤ ON THE MAT: The first time a yoga class completely held my attention was in St. Louis. It was my first-ever Vinyasa, and it wasn't that I was trying to accomplish dharana—it just sort of happened. I felt myself mesmerized by the new movements, the pace of the class, the puzzle pieces of putting together each flow—I was completely devouring each morsel of class. When in yoga, the opposite of dharana happens for us sometimes. We distract ourselves from the class because it's too hard, or slower-paced than what we expected, or we have a lot going on in our lives and can't pull ourselves away from our daily problems. By focusing on exactly what's in front of us, we dissolve inner conflict and open our minds to the next limb, dhyana.

SEVENTH LIMB: DHYANA—DEVOTION, MEDITATION

Dhyana is a combination of several of the principles we've discussed so far. This seventh limb begins the process of knitting together physical posture, breath control, control of senses, and concentration. Throughout class, you place each stepping stone in front of you to reach your final destination, samadhi. Dhyana is the last stone you place down in order to create your path. While everlasting bliss may not be a state found on Earth, meditation can provide some consolation by allowing us to focus on one thing with the intention of knowing its truth. Dhyana is usually referred to as meditation, but it's a different state most aligned with self-awareness and creating unity with a singular object.

❀ HOW TO PRACTICE IT EVERY DAY: The simplest and easiest way to bring meditation, particularly dhyana, into your every day could be starting your morning with gratitudes. Finding three things, big or small, that you're grateful for is a way to start each day with a moment of devotion toward positivity. Over time, you can add in a comfortable seat and five minutes of breathing. Then begin to add singular focus on breath and slowly increase the time you spend doing that. When beginning a meditation practice, you can start by dedicating it to anything: a person, a body part, maybe your whole self. You can add layers of intention to your meditation by including any of the practices we've discussed so far. Perhaps begin by just listening to your breath, then adding a search for stillness, then the principles of dhyana.

❀ ON THE MAT: Meditation in yoga, depending on what type, will only leave the end of class for you to melt away into dhyana. Be patient with yourself, as some days may be harder to come into a focused meditation. On others you may even fall completely asleep. The key to meditation post-yoga is finding your breath fully moving through the body, or even coming back to your mantra you set at the beginning of class.

EIGHTH LIMB:
SAMADHI

Drumroll, please! Samadhi is the final act: what we've all been waiting for. We've spent the last seven limbs analyzing, evaluating, reorganizing, letting go, opening up, and making space for Samadhi "bliss" or "enlightenment" to curl up in our lives. What's interesting about this last limb is that you're not all of a sudden swept away to a perfect place with zero stress, fuzzy slippers and martini in hand. Samadhi is about realizing that this life you have *is* perfect in its own way. Making yourself aware of your habits, imperfections, and negativity allows you to adjust what is in front of you to be that "blissful" life you seek. You've let go of fear, anger, and judgment, and you've put your ego on the shelf to make room in order to enjoy being present every moment of every day. Each limb builds off one another, but the last three are so important to find that sense of enlightenment.

❋ **HOW TO PRACTICE IT EVERY DAY:** Inevitably, no matter how many times I tell myself not to get frustrated, I still find anger budding during periods of stress. My inner tempo speeds up and my face gets warm, and I feel my chest constrict and fill with heat. We all fall back on old habits despite our best efforts to let them go and move forward. It happens—we're human. Just like my old habit of holding tension in my shoulders when my arms are extended to the sky in tree pose comes back; it happens, and that's okay. But when you gain self-awareness over time, you can remind yourself that the moment will pass, and that becoming angry or feeling negatively won't last. I remind myself that the late train will come, forgive myself for forgetting an umbrella on a rainy day, feel empathy for the slow-moving tourists who block my path. I remind myself to relax my shoulders on my exhale when I enter tree pose. We are all learning, we are all taking baby steps every day to be closer to our "higher selves" and in connection with our true inner selves.

Samadhi reminds us that the end destination doesn't matter, it's the journey. I can work for twenty years of my life at a job for a raise, but what did I *actually* do during those twenty years? What moments in my life brought joy to my heart? Where did my time go? Are most of my memories tied to my desk at work, or to spending time with the ones I loved? Was I able to take in the little moments: drinking coffee, smelling flowers, seeing a movie, soaking in beautiful sunny days? Did I find moments of relaxation and release of stress without worrying about the next fifty things on my to-do list? We get caught up in five-year plans and "end goals" that keep us from being present. Goals are good and having an idea of what you want in life is also great, but the eight limbs of yoga can help remind you day by day what is most important, what can be let go, and what you need more of. Each day will change for you, and sometimes you'll need more asteya or more sauca.

❀ **ON THE MAT:** A yoga class is a neatly wrapped gift placed in front of you. Yoga is not just flexibility or chanting *om*, it's not just holding a pose and moving to the next one. As you've come to find, we are looking toward finding our most full and whole selves. Finding unity within all aspects of who we are helps bring about peace and joy. Don't let your insecurities prevent you from fully letting your soul connect to your body during class.

I stumbled across an unattributed quote a year or so ago that resonated with me in the same way the limbs of yoga did:

> Don't overcomplicate life.
>
> Missing someone? Call them.
>
> Want to meet up? Invite.
>
> Want to be understood? Explain.
>
> Have questions? Ask.
>
> Don't like something? Say it.
>
> Like something? State it.
>
> Want something? Ask for it.
>
> Love someone? Tell them.
>
> We've only got one life; keep it simple.

I sometimes start classes off with this quote, explaining the ties between simplifying on the mat and carrying that simplification over into our personal lives. Fear of rejection, being told no, or fear of simply voicing an opinion can complicate normal and easy everyday interactions and relationships. In the same way, fear of falling out of a pose, or not being good enough to try a new pose, can happen during our practice. What happens when you simplify, focusing on your breath, committing to each pose 110 percent even if you fall over or look silly? Simplify. One of my clients came to class a week after I centered my class around the idea of simplifying. She told me about how she finally got the courage to ask for a raise as well as tell her lover her true feelings. A small shift in mindset can go a long way, whether it be on your mat, in your life, or both.

Though it may take time to open yourself up to the limbs of yoga, start with the basics of what you're looking to include in your practice. You've got new tools for your tool belt: different types of yoga and limbs of yogic philosophy. These can help build your personalized practice.

❊ 6 ❊

THE
ASANAS

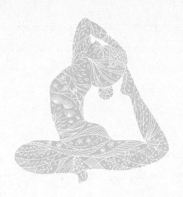

"Remember, it doesn't matter how deep into a posture you go,
what does matter is who you are when you get there."

—MAX STROM

LTHOUGH THIS WAS MENTIONED IN OUR DIS-
cussion of one of the limbs of yoga, I wanted to give you
an entire section on poses. So, whip out your tool belt
again, friends—I've got some good ones for you. If you've gotten this
far, it's pretty obvious that the poses are important. There are many
different names for yoga poses, some that may be familiar to you and
some less so. Even now, after practicing for years as well as teaching,
I will attend a class where my version of low lunge is completely different than what's being cued. When I was first beginning yoga, the
Sanskrit names caused panic when I couldn't remember exactly what

that pose was. Each teacher has their preference—you'll find a wide variety of instructors, some of whom will include Sanskrit and some won't. It doesn't mean anyone is right or wrong; what's important is correct alignment and cuing.

Curious about the meaning of some of the names? They range from the names of Hindu heroes, saints, and mythological creatures to names for animals, plants, and meteorological phenomena. There are many different spellings, which lead to different pronunciations—for example, savasana vs. shavasana. There isn't a "right" or "wrong" way, but the variety of naming conventions can get a little confusing. Some instructors even use contemporary names for poses, like "wild thing," which is like a flipped tabletop. From downward dog, lift your right leg to the sky into three-legged dog. Then begin to bend the knee, opening up the hip. As you open the hip, lift and twist the front of the body to the sky as you allow your right foot to fall behind you. With both feet now on the ground, the right arm is extended up and back. It's a great transition post as part of a Vinyasa flow or toward the end of class to really open up the hips.

I recently attended a class at Laughing Lotus NYC that included a pose called "OMG" (seriously!). It added a breath of fresh air into my practice—I was honestly on the edge of my seat since all of the poses were suddenly unfamiliar to me. There's something to be said for a modern take on yoga, and how it can be beneficial to this ancient, respected, and beloved practice. How do we keep poses traditional, yet adaptive to the times ahead? If renaming them proves to be a way to unite the mind, body, and spirit, create alignment, and allow the body to move in a way that is inspirational and open, who's to say it's incorrect?

While teaching aerial yoga, I began to name poses according to how they made me feel. My students got attached to many, like "Moon Goddess" and "Floating Mermaid," that they began to reject the original term or "correct" name in favor of feeling connected with the mystical, magical definition that their soul and body felt. That is what makes your practice worth it—your connection to the asana. If Sanskrit is what nourishes that connection, let it fly! If you like "corpse pose" instead of "savasana," live your best life. So finally, I give you a small slice of yoga asanas that you can refine on your own or in class. I've included the Sanskrit and the traditional English name. Which one you hear will depend on your studio or teachers. Names will vary, but over time you'll begin to recognize the term and pose with or without Sanskrit.

CHILD'S POSE | BALASANA

HOW TO DO IT: Start on all fours or on knees, big toes together, knees apart. Lay your torso between your thighs. Rest your head on the mat. Extend your arms forward.

MODIFICATION: Place block or blanket under tailbone for support or to close the gap. Close knees to rest belly on the thighs.

WHAT SHOULD I BE FEELING? Checking in with the hips, pose of rest.

Child's pose is the go-to pose throughout class. Modification is a sign of wisdom. When your body is craving rest throughout class, come back to child's pose. Reground, recoup, take a few breath cycles, then get back in the game. The hips might begin to feel tender if in this pose for a long time, so use your props when you need to! Make this pose active by pressing the hands into the mat while drawing the tailbone toward the heels.

ALL FOURS | BHARMANASANA

HOW TO DO IT: Come to a tabletop position with your hands, knees, and tops of feet making contact with the mat. Position your shoulders on top of your wrists, hips over knees, toes in line with knees, and all fingers pressed evenly.

MODIFICATION: Blanket under knees for support.

WHAT SHOULD I BE FEELING? Support of the spine, realignment of the spine.

BENEFITS: This pose is great for transitioning from the outside world into full yoga mode. Tabletop is the foundation of beginning class. Feeling the points of contact—hands, knees, tops of toes—brings about a sense of groundedness.

CAT/COW | MARJARYASANA/BITILASANA

HOW TO DO IT (CAT): Start on all fours. Inhale. Drop your belly. Tilt your pelvis. Set your gaze toward the sky.

HOW TO DO IT (COW): Start on all fours. Exhale. Curve your spine upward. Scoop your tailbone under. Set your gaze toward your navel, resting chin on chest.

MODIFICATION: Blanket under knees

WHAT SHOULD I BE FEELING? Elongation of the spine, flexion of the spine.

BENEFITS: This is a huge stress reliever! If I have some space before my acting auditions, I'll sneak away and go through cat/cow a few times. Syncing my breath and moving through both poses helps calm my nerves and feels so very good on my lower back. If you've got sciatica pain like me, this pose is definitely for you. Pro tip: Ladies, if you've got intense menstrual cramps, this pose is your friend (along with child's pose).

DOWNDOG | ADHO MUKHA SVANASANA

HOW TO DO IT: Start on all fours. Curl your toes under. Lift your hips to the sky. Press your arms back to be in line with your ears. Keep a soft bend in the knees. Lift heels to start. Gaze to your feet.

MODIFICATION: Keep knees bent throughout class.

WHAT SHOULD I BE FEELING? Elongation of the spine, shoulders wrapping back and down, hamstring stretch.

BENEFITS: This is THE POSE most people associate with yoga, and for good reason. There are so many lovely, delicious aspects to this asana. It opens the backs of the legs (runners, where you at?). This pose will lengthen without strain on any other part of the body. With how much we walk on a day-to-day basis, going up stairs, sitting for long periods of time, we don't think to give extra love to our hammies. It also elongates the spine and opens the chest, all while strengthening the arms. Magic, right?

MOUNTAIN POSE | TADASANA

HOW TO DO IT: Stand tall with your feet together. Distribute your weight evenly between left and right feet. Inhale, reaching arms overhead.

MODIFICATION: Keep arms by your side.

WHAT SHOULD I BE FEELING? Groundedness, long spine, even weight distribution.

BENEFITS: Okay, I know this one seems too simple. But that's the beauty of what yoga is! Working from the ground up, feet are rooted, soft bend the knees, neutral pelvis, shoulders relaxed, and heart space opened wide brings about confidence.

PLANK | KUMBHAKASANA

HOW TO DO IT: From downdog, roll forward to a plank position. Shoulders should be stacked on top of wrists, feet hips-width distance apart and grounding through base of toes. Actively press your heels toward the back of the room. Press up through the space between your shoulders. Gaze to the mat.

MODIFICATION: Come to knees.

WHAT SHOULD I BE FEELING? Hips aligned, core engaged, external rotation in shoulders to activate arm strength.

BENEFITS: Many of us have a memory of doing these sometime in elementary school PE class, waiting for the timer to end, then collapsing to the ground with exhaustion. I'm here to banish that memory and invite a new one in! This pose is major for toning the arms, abs, and glutes, and it strengthens muscles around the spine and helps with chaturanga prep. The key to a solid plank is to imagine pressing up through the space between the shoulders, as if you're pushing the ground away from you.

LOW PUSH-UP | CHATURANGA

HOW TO DO IT: From plank position, bend your elbows. Lower your body all at once. Begin to shift your weight forward.

MODIFICATION: Come to knees.

WHAT SHOULD I BE FEELING? Elbows gluing in toward the side body, core tight and engaged.

BENEFITS: I swear, this was one of the most difficult yoga poses for me to wrap my head around, but once accomplished correctly it feels SO GOOD. I see many clients with their elbows flying out to the side, which makes this pose nearly impossible. Practice coming into your low push-up and holding for a solid ten counts to build body awareness and strength. Hover one inch and hold, making sure you're still breathing, then you'll press up into the next pose.

UPWARD-FACING DOG | URDHVA MUKHA SVANASANA

HOW TO DO IT: Start facedown, with your forehead on the mat and hands directly under shoulders. Squeeze your glutes. Press through your hands. Roll your shoulders back and down. Reach your chest up and toward the wall.

MODIFICATION: Baby cobra—keep tops of feet pressing into mat as shoulders roll back and down, lifting chest off mat.

WHAT SHOULD I BE FEELING? Heart opening, drawing down from the armpits, not sinking into the shoulders.

BENEFITS: This pose is a huge spine strengthener. Working through baby cobra first, you'll begin to feel your back muscles stretch and strengthen over time. My lower back used to disagree with upward-facing dog, but by finding my right alignment, I feel my hips release and sciatica pain decrease. It also tones the butt combined with your Vinyasa flow—just saying.

ONE-LEGGED DOG | EKA PADA ADHO MUKHA SVANASANA

HOW TO DO IT: Start in downdog, with hips squared. Extend one leg up and back. Push your heel to the sky, toes pointing down. Continue to press evenly between left and right hands while keeping hips squared.

MODIFICATION: Only extend leg a little, an inch or two off the ground.

WHAT SHOULD I BE FEELING? Hips opening, hamstring stretch.

BENEFITS: Keeping the arms stable while extending your leg to the sky builds up so much muscle in the core, side body, and hamstring. You'll start to notice if one arm takes more weight than the other, and you'll find that over time things begin to even out. That heavy purse you carry on one shoulder instead of the other has more strength, and with one-legged dog, you're able to identify where these small imbalances are. It's a good prep for warrior 3, using your hands to steady you as you focus on squaring the hips while extending the leg. You want to feel as though your foot is pressing toward the space where the wall meets the ceiling.

RUNNER'S LUNGE | ARDHA HANUMANASANA

HOW TO DO IT: Start in plank or one-legged dog position. Step your foot in between hands. Line up the right knee over the ankle. Feel back heel pressing toward the back wall.

MODIFICATION: Place hands on blocks, or drop the back knee.

WHAT SHOULD I BE FEELING? Inner thighs on fire, big stretch on back-leg hamstring!

BENEFITS: Once I felt comfortable in this pose, my warrior series greatly improved. Tracking the right knee over the ankle while lengthening in the side body and feeling the back leg long, I realized how strong a foundation for my other poses this was. It's usually skipped over, or a transition pose. If you're able to spend some breath cycles refining in this shape, you'll find yourself benefiting later on in class. It also increases flexibility, as you activate the back leg while keeping the right knee aligned. Get ready for a deep, juicy stretch in those hip flexors!

LOW LUNGE | ANJANEYASANA

HOW TO DO IT: Drop your back knee to the mat. Crawl your front foot one inch forward. Start to feel the push of your hips toward the mat. Sweep your arms up to the sky. Relax your shoulders.

MODIFICATION: Keep hands on front thigh, pushing hands down to open collarbones.

WHAT SHOULD I BE FEELING? A continual stretch through inner thighs.

BENEFITS: While strengthening and stretching the legs, you also find incredible length in your side body and spine. When doing this correctly, it should be the most delectable. I mean it—this is one of my favorite poses. The right knee is over the ankle providing support as the hips stay square, stretching toward the mat as the arms extend to the sky. You're pushing and pulling to achieve maximum length throughout the body. Low lunge releases tension in your hips while strengthening your hamstrings and knees, all while building mental focus! The biggest problem I see in my students is in getting their knees to go over the toes, keeping them in check. There should not be ANY pressure directly on your back knee. If you're feeling this, scoot those front toes forward more to make space for your hips to release more toward the mat.

HIGH LUNGE | UTTHITA ASHWA SANCHALANASANA

HOW TO DO IT: Start in runner's lunge position. Tuck your back toes. Check your front knee alignment. Engage your core, raising your arms up overhead. Keep hips squared to front. The back heel should push toward the back of the room on the base of the toe. Shoulders are relaxed.

MODIFICATION: Shorten stance.

WHAT SHOULD I BE FEELING? Hips in alignment, core engaged, push and pull of hips.

BENEFITS: Once I became friends with high lunge, my practice completely shifted. At the beginnings of my yoga certification, I remember dreading whenever my instructor cued into it. My body rejected this pose and I simply didn't understand its use. Activating the back foot is KEY. As soon as I lifted up onto the base of my toes and pressed my heel as if I were stamping it against the back of the room, I felt space created for my hips to align, along with feeling control over my front knee while stretching through the groin. Through high lunge, I was able to deepen my warrior series.

WARRIOR 2 | VIRABHADRASANA II

HOW TO DO IT: Starting position can vary, but you can begin from high lunge position. Seal your back foot down while keeping your front knee aligned. Open arms wide to T shape. Gaze over your front fingers. Front knee should cover up the baby toes, finding external rotation; all you should see is your big toe. Keep your back arm aligned with the front. Your hips should be in line with the ribcage, aligned with the shoulders. Release the clenching in your glutes. Equalize your weight distribution between both feet.

MODIFICATION: Shorten stance.

WHAT SHOULD I BE FEELING? Inner thigh engagement, stretch along side bodies, like someone's pulling you from the front and back of room, like your heels are moving toward each other.

BENEFIT: A major benefit of warrior 2 is increased stamina. This was another pose that didn't make sense to me for a long, long time. I always felt a pull in my hips, and it hurt my IT band on my right side. With properly cued alignment from a fabulous teacher, something clicked in my brain and my body followed. I see a lot of my clients squeezing their glutes to hold them in this pose, when really that's preventing you from going deeper. You're also stretching and strengthening your ankles, wrists, groins, lungs, shoulders—all of it. This pose was named after a warrior (Virabhadra) who, in many tales, is painted as a tiger-skin-wearing, club-wielding warrior with thousands of eyes, feet, and heads protecting the innocent. So the next time you're cued into this pose, take up space, feel the righteousness of this fierce warrior.

PEACEFUL WARRIOR | SHANTI VIRABHADRASANA

HOW TO DO IT: From warrior 2, keep your legs exactly where they are—with front knee aligned over ankle and back foot sealed down as the inner thighs are activated. Flip your front palm, carving through space toward the sky. Continually push through your hips. Pull through your hand and fingers. Create space between your vertebrae.

MODIFICATION: Keep back hand on the thigh for support; over time you can add a bind.

WHAT SHOULD I BE FEELING? Stretch along side body.

BENEFIT: This strengthens the legs while also lengthening

your side body. I always describe any time you are reaching behind, for a backbend, side angle, etc., that you want to think about growing tall like a sunflower, then letting your own weight guide you down. There's always a sense of life and reach instead of just reaching back. Peaceful warrior relieves back pain, while opening the torso for deeper breathing.

EXTENDED SIDE ANGLE | UTTHITA PARSVAKONASANA

HOW TO DO IT: (Transition from peaceful warrior) Front forearm comes to top of your thigh. The back arm extends up overhead. Roll your back shoulder away. Set your gaze to the sky. For a deeper stretch, lengthen front arm to the ground.

MODIFICATION: Shorten stance, keep arm extended to sky.

WHAT SHOULD I BE FEELING? Fire in front thigh, stretch from back foot all the way to fingertips.

BENEFIT: I've found there's much core strength involved with extended side angle, but this pose truly works the whole body out. It strengthens the inner thighs, lengthens the side body, and tones the core. It's also therapeutic for constipation, sciatica pain, and back pain. I tell my students to imagine they're putting on a corset, to keep the core strong and side body lengthened.

CHAIR POSE | UTKATASANA

HOW TO DO IT: Start with centerlined feet, big toes together, and inner ankle bones and inner knees all closed tightly, as if trying to hold a piece of paper between them. Ground down through ball of foot and heel. Bend the knees. Hinge at the hips. Sit your hips back while making sure you can see your toes. Don't tilt your pelvis. Extend arms up overhead. For extra spice, lift the heels while keeping depth in your hips.

MODIFICATION: Keep hands in active prayer at heart center; use a wall to support the spine.

WHAT SHOULD I BE FEELING? Fired-up thighs, core engaged.

BENEFITS: I've seen it all when it comes to this pose. Many will immediately sit as low as possible, but my trick to chair is to slowly work your way into it. Once you get the first few steps out of the way, before sitting back as far as possible, check your form. Make sure you can see your toes, feel the shoulders engaged, then add the arms and begin to sit back. There's unfortunately no prize for the person who sits the lowest first, so take your time placing each brick. Chair pose will tone your legs like crazy, but it requires your core to be engaged as well.

TREE | VRKSASANA

HOW TO DO IT: Starting in mountain position, ground down through one foot. Lift the opposite heel. Find the external rotation in your leg. Draw your toes up the inner leg line, pressurizing above or below the knee. Keep your two hips in one line. Hands extend overhead. Root (pun intended) down through standing leg.

MODIFICATION: Keep toes on mat, heel pressing into standing leg, or hands stay in prayer.

WHAT SHOULD I BE FEELING? Balance pose, energy in standing leg, and support from balancing leg.

BENEFITS: Tree pose challenges our balance. I feel this pose is also one of those "classic yoga poses" you see in commercials or on social media as THE pose to do. When done correctly, there are some major gains to be had. Pay attention to your toes next time you're in tree. Notice if they habitually want to grip the mat. What can you do to feel yourself pushing through the mat while also finding expansion in the spine, reaching the hands to the sky? I thought for a long time that it was about holding your foot up, when really that foot is essential to the push and pull of this pose. Over time, challenge yourself even more by closing your eyes and relaxing all tension in the face to center yourself. This is a great pose to come into before an interview, first date, audition . . . any situation in which you'd normally be anxious.

Tree pose plus pranayama can help ground and center you. Something about being able to stand confidently on one foot with your eyes closed can bring a sense of peace to a day where nervous energy is present.

WARRIOR 3 | VIRABHADRASANA III

HOW TO DO IT: Starting position can vary, but from tree pose, continue to ground down through standing leg. Similar to one-legged dog, keep hips square as you shift your moving leg behind you. Hips stay aligned. Keep heel to the sky with toes pointed down. Hands stay in in prayer, extended overhead or framing the body.

MODIFICATION: Take hands to blocks.

WHAT SHOULD I BE FEELING? Balance pose, full body engaged, length in spine, energy pulling from crown of head, energy pushing from back foot.

BENEFITS: Warrior 3 can be extremely frustrating at times, so be patient with yourself! Again, no prizes in yoga for highest leg, so work on squaring your hips first, then lifting the back leg higher over time. Warrior 3 is a major core toner. Squaring your hips takes quite a bit of body awareness and engagement of the obliques and core. When the arms are engaged properly, you'll feel soreness the next day. Play with variations: Arms reached over head with shoulders pulling back and down and palms rotated toward each other, hands in activated prayer, or arms framing the body like an airplane.

BRIDGE | SETU BANDHA SARVANGASANA

HOW TO DO IT: On your back, take your feet to the mat at hips-width distance. Brush the backs of your heels with your fingers. Press your hands into the mat. Lift your hips to the sky. Interlace your fingers behind back.

MODIFICATION: Place block underneath sacrum, keep hips down.

WHAT SHOULD I BE FEELING? Hips lifted, stretch along the spine.

BENEFITS: Bridge pose is extremely important, and I do my best to include this in every single yoga class I instruct. Bridge stretches the neck, back, and spine while calming the mind, alleviating stress, and soothing tummy digestion, while stimulating the lungs and organs. Remember to breathe; I notice a lot of my students holding their breath in this pose. Bridge pose will help build to a full wheel—an advanced progression of bridge, where the palms are flipped down and the hips are extended toward the sky.

HALF MOON | ARDHA CHANDRASANA

HOW TO DO IT: From warrior 2, push down through your front right foot as you lift the back leg to the sky. Front hand will come to the ground at the top of the mat; back arm will extend to the sky. Top hip is stacking on top of standing leg as you feel your standing leg rooting down into the mat. Allow your torso to open up toward the sky, while keeping your shoulders in one line. Back foot is flexed, leg is parallel to the floor (or as close to parallel as you can get!) Gaze is on the ground ahead of you. Spicy option: set gaze to your extended hand toward the sky.

MODIFICATION: Hand on the ground can come to a block, hand to the sky can come to the hip. Keep gaze forward.

WHAT SHOULD I BE FEELING? Your body lengthening from earth to sky, and your core muscles strengthening.

BENEFITS: I try to stray away from favorite poses, but this one makes me feel like I'm FLYING. There's something so freeing about half moon, and this pose really captures "push and pull." This pose strengthens your ankles, legs, gluten, and abs while also stretching and expanding the hamstrings. Half moon can help with digestion and anxiety. There's something so satisfying about rooting down through your standing leg, while the top arm and leg are lengthening, opening, and reaching away. Feel the back foot energized, allow yourself to expand through every limb of the body. Balancing poses can be intimidating, but know that with time and control they get easier. Be patient, use your props, and feel your breath ground you. If you fall out of it and fail, great. This is building body awareness.

MOVING AND BREATHING

Now we have the poses, we have the breath . . . how do we connect the two? Through my training at Studio ANYA in Manhattan, I was able to truly connect my breath and body. For years, I did yoga without that piece of the puzzle. I didn't understand when to breathe. Occasionally I had instructors cue it, but for whatever reason it wouldn't stick. I felt no movement in class—I would hold the pose, move to the next one. Once I was introduced to push and pull, the clouds parted.

Refining each pose is so important: finding your hips aligned, your shoulders relaxed, your knee over your ankle . . . there are so many elements to each pose, and bringing pranayama along with it is essential. Any time you find a push in a pose, it connects to your exhale. Any time you are pulling, you should find your inhale. Different yoga styles will have different pranayamas and where to put the inhale and exhale will vary. For Vinyasa in particular, in all my years of practice . . . this has been the most useful. So don't overlook it!

❖ 7 ❖

LET'S FLOW

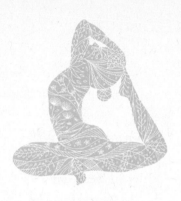

"Yoga does not remove us from the responsibilities of our everyday life, but rather places our feet firmly and resolutely in the practical ground of experience. We don't transcend our lives; we return to the life we left behind in hopes of something better."

—DONNA FARHI

I'VE PUT TOGETHER SOME FLOWS FOR YOU TO DO ON your own, outside of the yoga classroom. There are so many excuses we come up with to avoid adding yoga to our days, and not getting to class is number one. Even as an instructor, it's tempting to find excuses not to take a few minutes out of my day. Here are some ways to suck it up, toss your mat down in even a very limited space, and play.

BEGINNER FLOW

1. **CHILD'S POSE:** Start in child's pose, observing your body, tapping fingers on the mat, checking in. Five breath cycles here, then move on.

2. **ALL FOURS:** Finding your tabletop position, check all points of contact: hands, knees, tops of feet. Press evenly between them all for five breath cycles.

3. **DOWNDOG:** Tuck the toes and press into downdog. Check alignment of hands and feet. Keep a soft bend in your knees as you notice your spine. Gently lower knees down to the mat.

4. **TAKE THIS MINI FLOW 5 TO 10 TIMES.** Inhale to all fours, exhale to downdog, inhale knees to mat, exhale child's pose. (A sequence from my yoga certification with ANYA that is my ALL-TIME favorite way to get warmed up.)

MORNING FLOW | SUN SALUTATION

1. **MOUNTAIN POSE:** To begin, stand straight and tall. Take a moment of gratitude for the upcoming day. When beginning my morning with yoga, I like to set some sort of intention of what I'd like to receive that day. Maybe that is joy, encouragement, silence, stillness—whatever meets your needs. Inhale your arms up overhead.

2. **FORWARD FOLD:** Exhale, sweep arms down. Keep hands and gaze ahead of you. Toward the later flows when you are more flexible in this sun salutation (the seventh or eighth repetition), grab the backs of the ankles and release the head.

3. **STANDING FORWARD BEND:** Inhale and come up halfway, placing hands on the shins. You should feel length in the spine as well as the hamstrings.

4. **PLANK:** As you inhale, step back one foot at a time to your high plank pose. Shift the weight forward as you lower down into a low push-up on the exhale.

5. **UPWARD-FACING DOG:** Inhale, keeping the elbows close to the sides of the body as you pull the heart space up and forward. Fully engage the legs as you roll the shoulders back and down.

6. **DOWNWARD DOG:** Exhale as you press your hips toward the sky. Ground down through the hands and take one breath cycle. Inhale; walk four steps to the top of the mat.

7. **STANDING FORWARD FOLD:** Inhale and come up halfway. Exhale, fold forward.

8. **UPWARD SALUTE/REVERSE SWAN DIVE:** Sweep the arms up toward the sky on your inhale. Exhale arms to prayer.

9. **MOUNTAIN POSE:** Inhale/exhale with hands by your side or in prayer.

10. **REPEAT THIS CYCLE 20 TO 25 TIMES,** ending with a brief savasana or five-minute sitting meditation. This sequence

always gets my blood flowing and breath regulated and wakes me up almost as much as a cup of coffee.

OFFICE FLOW | 10-MINUTE SEQUENCE

When you need a quick little wake-up sesh between meetings, or any time when you're short on time, here are a few quick poses to rejuvenate your body and mind.

1. CHILD'S POSE: Spend five to ten breath cycles here. Let your head rock side to side, heavy exhales.
2. ALL FOURS (CAT/COW): Take your time moving through these poses, noticing the spine, connecting the inhale to cow, exhale to cat.
3. THREAD THE NEEDLE: From all fours, inhale right arm to the sky. Exhale, take the right arm in between the left arm and thigh. Right shoulder and ear come to the mat. Left arm extends over head on the mat. Take five to ten breath cycles. Repeat on the other side.
4. DOWNWARD DOG: Come into your downdog. Pedal it out, shake the head yes/no, yawn/sigh. Take ten to twenty breath cycles.
5. MOUNTAIN POSE: From downdog, slowly walk all the way up to the top of the mat. Roll up, bone by bone; head arrives last. Bring your hands to your side for three full breath cycles.

NIGHTTIME FLOW

Insomnia kicking in? Having a rough time falling asleep? Here's a quick flow to help with restlessness. Take your time and stay in each pose longer than you think you might need to. Breath is key!

1. CHILD'S POSE: Using a blanket or block between your heels/tailbone, come into child's pose. Let your breath be minimum four counts for the inhale and exhale.

2. DOWNWARD DOG: Shifting the weight forward, move through all fours and into your dog. Inhale the right leg to the sky, stepping it to the outside of the right foot.

3. HAPPY BABY: Coming on to your back, bring the knees into the chest. Separate the knees away from the rib cage, taking the hands to the outside edges of the feet, or use your peace fingers grab for the big toes. If not accessible, take the hands to the knees. Keep the feet aligned with the knees as you begin to gently push the feet into the hands, while pulling the hands down toward the feet. Allow the body to rock side to side. Spend a full minute here, noticing your breath.

4. SINGLE LEG TO CHEST: From happy baby, draw the right knee into the chest, using your lower abdominal gently take the left leg long in front of you. Let the left leg be heavy, as you flex both feet. Interlace the fingers below the right knee as you melt your shoulders into the mat. Keep hips in line, breath steady. Option to extend right leg toward the sky for

a deeper stretch. Another full minute or so here, keeping breath steady. Repeat on the other side.

5. BRIDGE POSE: Still supine, take both feet flat to the floor hips width distance. Allow your fingertips to reach the backs of the ankles. Begin to press your hands down into the mat as you take the hips toward the sky. Release any tension in the gluten, let your spine and hamstrings do the work. Squeeze the shoulder blades toward each other like you're grabbing a pencil between them, and interlace your fingers behind the back. Spend 30 seconds or so here, keeping your hips lifted. Modify by simply placing a block underneath the sacrum/ low back.

6. SUPINE TWIST: Come to lying fully on your back. Similar to single leg to chest, draw right leg in and extend the bottom leg. Shift more toward the center of your mat as you draw the right knee across to the left as you extend your right arm long. Set the gaze over the right finger tips as the left hand comes to the top of the right thigh for added stretch. Allow the right shoulder to melt into the mat as you relax your shoulders away from your ears. Send breath to the right side body. Stay for a full minute (or longer if it feels nice,) then repeat on the other side.

7. END WITH RECLINED BUTTERFLY: Slowly roll onto your back. Take the soles of the feet together; allow the knees to fall open. Add blocks under knees for support. Take one hand

to your heart, one hand to your belly and being to observe your breath. Take a full inhale for four counts, full exhale for four counts.

Reclined Butterfly | Supta Baddha Konasana

From downdog, gently come onto your knees and lay onto your back. Take the soles of the feet together, knees open wide. Use any props that feel necessary. Spend a full two minutes here.

TRAVEL FLOW

This flow is perfect for when you're on the road—in small hotel rooms with limited space, when you don't have a yoga mat, or any time when you want to get rid of the ickiness of a long car or airplane ride.

1. ALL FOURS (CAT/COW): Take several rounds of cat/cow on your own time, noticing your breath, feeling your hands grounding down into the floor/mat, moving at your own pace. Tuck the toes under and hover the knees one inch off of the mat for a count of ten. Lower knees down gently.

2. CHILD'S POSE: After your knee hover, press back into child's pose for a five to ten breath count. Feel the tailbone draw down toward the heels as you wiggle into this one. Notice your hips and if there is any tightness or stiffness. Inhale forward to all fours, exhale, and press back into child's pose. Repeat this ten times.

3. **DOWNWARD DOG:** Next, curl the toes (option for another ten-count knee hover) and press the hips back into downdog. Enjoy this! Especially when traveling, we feel tense all over the body. Pedal the feet out, shake the head yes and no, let out your biggest exhales. Hands press evenly, let the head be heavy. Ten breath cycles in downdog.

4. **RAGDOLL:** Inhale walking four steps up to the top of the mat, feet hips-width distance. Keep a soft bend in the knees as you grab for your opposite elbows and sway. Bounce the hips, bend the knees, let there be movement while the head is heavy and hips are hinged. Start rolling up bone by bone, letting your head come up last with a soft bend in your knees.

5. **MOUNTAIN:** You know this one! This is where we reground. Feel your feet underneath you, relax your shoulders, and spend ten to fifteen breaths here, observing your limbs and reconnecting with your body. Let go of the travel stress, open up to reconnecting. Inhale your arms up overhead, exhale to sweep arms down. Repeat ten times.

6. **FORWARD FOLD:** Take your hands all the way down to the mat using blocks if need be, soft bend in the knees, release the head and pedal it out like in downdog. Bounce the hips up and down (like a yoga twerk) and let out big exhales.

7. **PLANK:** Inhale, then step one foot at a time back into your plank. Once everything is lined up, hold for five breath cycles, continually pressing up through the space between

A LITTLE BIT OF YOGA

the shoulders. On your exhale, lower knees, chest, chin, and come into your baby cobra.

8. Take this flow five to ten times.

OPTIONAL: SPICE IT UP

To make this flow even more interesting, add:

1. HIGH LUNGE: Five breath cycles, refining this pose by keeping both hips in line, energy in the hands and back heel.

2. WARRIOR 2: From high lunge, seal back foot down, arms come down into a T shape, continually releasing any tension in your glutes and tracking your right knee. Set gaze over right fingertips as you use body awareness to bring the back arm in line with the front.

3. REVERSE WARRIOR: Keeping the legs where they are, flip the right palm up and back for five to ten breath cycles.

4. EXTENDED SIDE ANGLE: Again, legs stay there! Front forearm comes to the top of the thigh, back arm reaches up toward the sky then tips forward. Imagine you're wearing a corset and both side bodies are supported and lengthened.

5. REPEAT on each side.

❈ 8 ❧

MINDFULNESS TECHNIQUES

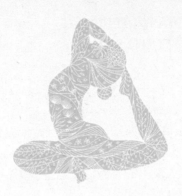

"When you own your breath, nobody can steal your peace."

—ANONYMOUS

ASIDE FROM A RIGOROUS, SWEAT-INDUCING flow, yoga can also be used simply for stretching, mindfulness meditation, or a combination of the two. We touched on Restorative yoga in the different types, but here are a few seated poses you can do outside of a flow in your own space, on your own time. Combining these poses with the breathing we covered earlier can help bring a sense of serenity to your day.

SEATED FORWARD FOLD |
PASCHIMOTTANASANA

HOW TO DO IT: Sit with your legs out long in front of you. Shimmy back and forth so you feel like you're sitting on your sit bones. Keep a soft bend in the knees as you reach up, then fold forward over your legs. Think of keeping your spine like a cow's back instead of a cat's back, letting the low belly fall on top of the thighs.

MODIFICATION: Bend your knees more, take a rolled blanket under your knees, separate your feet to protect the lower back.

WHAT SHOULD I BE FEELING? Stretch across the lower back/spine/hamstrings.

BENEFITS: This is a stretch I remember doing for years during volleyball practice, gym class, ballet, and any and every sport-related activity. I never really understood what this stretch was targeting; I just remember it was always something that happened after any kind of rigorous working out. The point of this pose is not to touch your toes. I could care less if you can reach them, you do not get any extra points or cookies for touching your toes. I want you to feel this in your spine and hamstrings with a major release in the head. Maybe this means you only reach your calves. As always, feel the lift first, then exhale and find the fold.

HEAD TO KNEE | JANU SIRASANA

HOW TO DO IT: From a comfortable seat position, take one leg to the side. Your opposite foot comes in to the inner thigh of the extended leg. Square your body to the extended leg as you lift up to fold forward, similar to the seated forward fold. Eventually the goal is to get your head to your knee . . . but take your time.

MODIFICATION: Use a strap around the extended foot; keep a soft bend in the knee to protect the lower back.

WHAT SHOULD I BE FEELING? Isolation stretching in the singular side of the body.

BENEFITS: This stretch is good for digestion while stretching the spine, groin, and hamstring. It can also help relieve mild depression. I love to follow seated forward fold with this on each side, as it feels like a way to deepen each side on its own. Feel yourself grounding down through both sit bones (aka the tail bone) as you keep the spine long. There are no prizes for touching your toes! Be aware of your lower back, and only fold as far forward as feels beneficial. Same as your forward fold, keep the spine like a cow back rather than a cat.

MARICHI POSE | MARICHYASANA

HOW TO DO IT: Start with both legs extended in front of you. Bend the right leg, placing the foot flat on the ground and as close to the sit bones as possible. Feel the heart space reaching forward, and feel as though someone is pulling you from the crown of your head. Begin to rotate toward the direction of your right leg. Take your left arm, creating a ninety-degree angle, and begin to hook it on the outside of your right knee. The right hand should press down behind you, close to your bum, helping you lift up and twist. Keep the left leg long and activated.

MODIFICATION: Sit on a blanket.

WHAT SHOULD I BE FEELING? Length in the spine, twisting from rib cage.

BENEFITS: Twisting poses feel like absolute magic when done properly. The key to this one is to continuously lift up; my favorite way to cue into this is "lift and twist," à la Harry Potter's "swish and flick," finding room in your vertebrae. As someone with major sciatica pain, this pose has helped me tremendously when I feel it flaring up. The farther the hand from the body, the less you get out of this pose. Keep it close, pressing down to pull up and twist.

BUTTERFLY | BADDHA KONASANA

HOW TO DO IT: Grounding down through your sit bones,
take your feet together, heels and toes touching. Knees
should then go wide, keeping hips open. Grab your ankles
with your hands and begin to fold forward, heart reaching
out. Only fold as far forward as your spine allows without
straining.

MODIFICATION: Add blocks under each of the knees.

WHAT SHOULD I BE FEELING? This is a major inner thigh
stretch, plus a stretch along the spine.

BENEFITS: What's so lovely about butterfly is that it
provides release to your lower back without your needing to
have super-flexible hamstrings. You're also releasing tension
in your shoulders and neck while folding forward. The
heavier you can make your head, the more release you'll find.

PIGEON | EKA PADA RAJAKAPOTASANA

HOW TO DO IT: From downdog, inhale your leg to
the sky and draw your shin across the mat. Do your best
to keep your hips squared. Untuck your back toes and
peek over your shoulder to check the alignment of your
back leg. Press your hands down into the mat, feeling as
if someone is pulling you up from the crown of your head.

Begin to slowly walk your hands forward, still keeping length in your spine. Rest your forehead on a block, your hands, or the mat. Arms should extend on the mat over the head.

MODIFICATION: This pose lends itself well to props. Add a blanket under the glute of the leg that's in front.

WHAT SHOULD I BE FEELING? A stretch in the hip flexors and hamstrings.

BENEFITS: Hip openers: It's a complicated relationship. I'm greeted with many wincing faces, groans of pain, and wiggly students while cueing this pose. I like to think of it as a deep-deep-tissue massage. It's silly to think about stretching for something as normal as walking or sitting, but over time those two simple activities build up tension in the hip flexors. That's where our good friend pigeon comes in! This pose will help release those tight hips, if you let yourself actually give in to it. The hardest part is finding stillness when your hips are screaming, "WHY DON'T YOU STRETCH ME OUT MORE?!" It's super important to keep your hips even in pigeon. Don't be afraid to load up on props, doing everything you can to maintain the alignment as you walk the hands forward. Next time you're in class, flag down an instructor and ask if everything looks good to go. (NEVER be afraid to ask for help during class!)

RECLINED BUTTERFLY | SUPTA BADA KANASANA

HOW TO DO IT: Lying on your back, bring the soles of your feet together to touch. Let your knees fall open wide. Notice where the low back/sacrum is, making sure there's no major arching in the spine.

MODIFICATION: Add blocks under each of the knees.

WHAT SHOULD I BE FEELING? This is a major inner thigh stretch.

BENEFITS: Within the first ten seconds of being in this pose, you will immediately regret every time you decided not to stretch after an intense workout. Reclined butterfly is an extremely intense stretch for the groin, and I will often start and end class with it. It's satisfying and it stimulates the heart while also improving circulation throughout the body.

❖ 9 ❖

CREATING A POSITIVE CHANGE IN YOUR LIFE

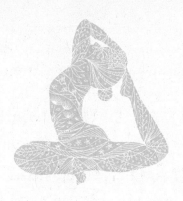

"Most people have no idea how good their body is designed to feel."
—KEVIN TRUDEAU

THROUGHOUT MY TIME AS A PRACTICING YOGI and as an instructor, my main goal has been to bring the practice of yoga into the lives of as many people as possible. There is room in the yoga world for anyone and everyone, and if that is something that has in any small way sparked your interest, but hesitation has followed, I hope this little book can nudge you back in the right direction. Even something as small as inviting a new pranayama into your mornings before you get ready, noticing how you physically stand in line at the grocery store, or observing your reactions to negative happenings in your life can ignite a whole different outlook. You may think that "yoga people"

113

sound crazy talking about it sometimes, and even I for a while couldn't fully get on board with the assumed "yoga lifestyle." But the more you study and practice yoga, the closer you will come to finding the yoga that works for YOU. Try different types of yoga during different periods of your life, and be open to reinvestigating it as your path changes.

IT DOESN'T HAPPEN OVERNIGHT

Like anything good in life, yoga takes time. You will not be a well-balanced, healthy-eating warrior 3 champion after one class. Though it may seem intimidating, give a few studios a try, and make sure you try out classes in the different styles outlined in this book. Think of it like sampling cakes before your wedding. You may want the vanilla with buttercream, but when you try the German chocolate, it might unexpectedly be the right thing for you. I bounced around many studios before I found one that fit. That changes every few years, as does my practice. It's important to find a studio you love, as well as an instructor that makes you want to come back over and over again. Bring a friend with you if you feel weird going alone. If you know class settings aren't your thing, try a few flows from the earlier chapters, then begin to do a little online research for videos to follow in your own home. Treat yourself to a new yoga mat and blocks and make your space available to practice.

Now that you've got a tool belt stocked with the essentials to get yoga into your life, use it well. The more good you do for yourself, the more you'll notice how it affects not only you but the people in your life, your workplace, and the world in general. The closer you gravitate toward your inner truth and most authentic version of who you are, the clearer your perspective on life will be, and that will have a real impact. There's no perfect cure for being upset, no Band-Aid for bad news, and no all-encompassing recipe to fix feeling crummy . . . but you can breathe. Connecting your body to your inhale and exhale, simplifying what it is to be alive, and listening to what you really need are all ways to mend the negativity in your life.

ACKNOWLEDGMENTS

I dedicate this book to anybody who's ever passed by a yoga class and thought, "WOW, I could never do something like that." If you told chubby, eighth-grade me that I'd one day be writing a book about yoga, I would have been extremely confused and immediately asked, "What is yoga . . . ?" I was never physically fit growing up; I was never flexible or strong. I was easily embarrassed, shy, and insecure. Yoga was the first real introduction to fitness that intrigued me, and I didn't find it until I was seventeen. It's never too late to begin a new passion or hobby—allow yourself to be unafraid of a new beginning.

Thank you to my parents and brother for never questioning when I tell them about a new acting, yoga, or photography project, and for always supporting me before even asking exactly what it entails. To Ryan Montgomery, for listening to me consistently gush about yoga on the daily, coming to take my classes as often as possible, and playing me my favorite songs on his acoustic guitar while I spent hours of our time together writing this book. Finally, to Nicole Lara, who suggested my name for this endeavor. She, without skipping a beat, assured me this book was mine and believed in me 100 percent. And of course, to Kate Zimmermann for being there every single step of the way with encouraging words.

ABOUT THE AUTHOR

Meagan Stevenson hails from San Antonio, Texas, and made her move to New York City after earning a BFA in Acting from Webster University's Conservatory of Theatre Arts in St. Louis, Missouri. While there, she discovered a love of yoga, dance, and aerial performance that, when combined with her thirst for knowledge and natural Texan tenacity, led her to pursue these art forms professionally when she arrived in the city. Along with her 200hr yoga certification from Studio ANYA, she has two Aerial yoga certifications, is Schwinn certified, and Lyra certified through Cirqufit. Aside from teaching yoga in the city, she's also the Operations Coordinator as well as yoga instructor for hOM, a company that brings yoga into residential and commercial buildings. She enjoys empowering others, and helping people find the beauty and peace within themselves, and when she's not doing that on a mat or hanging from aerial silks, she's doing it from behind a camera as a professional photographer or over a plate of cookies as a recreational baker.

Find her at: wwwmeaganstevenson.com;
on Instagram (@meaganstevenson25);
and on Twitter (MeaganLeigh14).

INDEX